CAESAREAN
RECOVERY

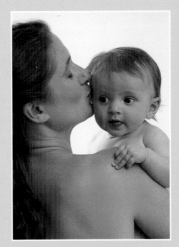

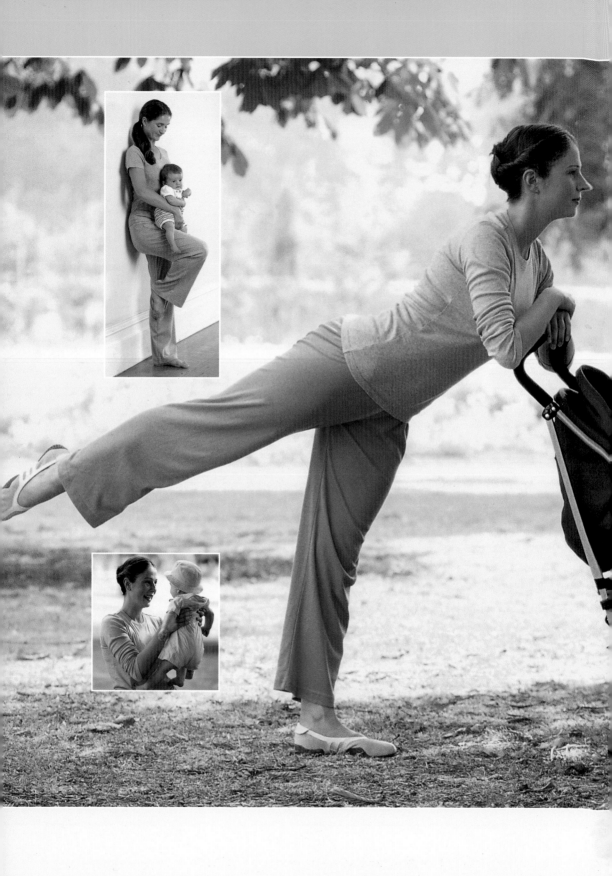

CAESAREAN
RECOVERY

CHRISSIE GALLAGHER-MUNDY

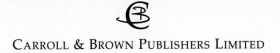

CARROLL & BROWN PUBLISHERS LIMITED

Revised edition first published Autumn 2010

First published in 2004 in the United Kingdom by
Carroll & Brown Publishers Limited
20 Lonsdale Road
London NW6 6RD

A CIP catalogue record for this book is available from the British Library

ISBN 978-1-907952-06-7

10987654321

Printed and bound in China

*Publisher's note: the information contained in this book should be used as a
general reference guide and does not constitute, and is not intended to substitute
for, an expert's medical advice or legal advice. Consult your doctor or healthcare
professional prior to following any treatment or exercises contained in this book.*

Contents

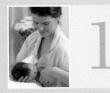
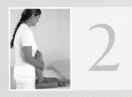
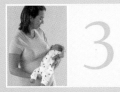
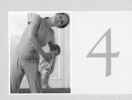
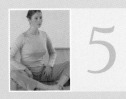

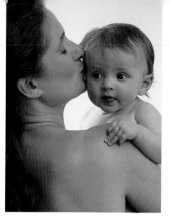

Introduction

Most of you reading this book know that your babies are going to be delivered by elective caesarean section. Some of you, however, will have planned for a vaginal delivery but circumstances at the time necessitated a surgical delivery. But whether you knew ahead of time or found out after the fact, all of you should find this book a valuable aid to a complete and problem-free recovery.

A lifesaving operation for baby and mother

Although the caesarean section has been part of human culture since ancient times, it used always to be considered a very last resort to try to save the baby rather than to preserve the mother's life. It wasn't until the nineteenth century that the medical profession started to consider the possibility that the operation could be used to save both mother and child. Gradually the caesarean, although still seen as a last resort, began to be used more frequently and with greater success. Today the operation has become more commonplace, with around 25 percent of British mothers giving birth by caesarean section.

There are several important reasons why a caesarean might be considered necessary, and these are discussed later in the book. If you have (or had) been offered an elective cesarean, your doctor should have explained to you and your birth partner why the operation is thought to be necessary, and he or she should answer any questions you may have before you sign a consent form. However, in the event of an emergency caesarean, there may not be time to have a detailed discussion, and you may feel as though you're being pressured into agreeing to the decision. In such a case it helps to remember that you will only be offered a caesarean if it is considered necessary for your health and for the safe birth of your baby.

Major surgery

It's important to realise that when you have a caesarean section you are having major abdominal surgery. A caesarean birth puts greater demands on your body and its recovery than if you have a vaginal delivery. Although any pain will be managed in hospital, there are other items that will help relieve discomfort, such as a maternity belt to support your scar, which you may want to include in your hospital bag. Your stay in the hospital will be a few days longer than if you have a straightforward vaginal birth, so you may want to take this into account when you are packing for your hospital stay.

If you plan to breastfeed there are special breastfeeding positions that will make feeding easier for you (see pages 26–29). Finding out about these before the delivery could be helpful. Getting useful tips from other moms, too, will make your stay in hospital a more pleasant experience.

Once you're home

All new mothers have to learn to adjust to life with a newborn, but also you will be recovering from major abdominal surgery. It can take up to six months before your incision fully heals, and even after it has healed you can expect to feel some numbness in the area until your nerves have a chance to regenerate, sometimes up to three months after the delivery.

Try to rest as much as possible during the first few weeks at home. The more rest you allow yourself during the initial recovery period, the faster your recuperation will be. It will take time for your abdominal muscles to regain their strength and flexibility.

Getting back into shape

Gentle exercise is important in order to facilitate healing of the muscles. Although you are unlikely to feel that you want to exercise immediately after the birth, it will be helpful to get up and start moving around as soon as the effects of the anaesthetic have worn off. On pages 38–43, you will find some simple exercises you can do while lying in bed, which are the first steps on your road to recovery. From these initial steps, as you become stronger, you will gradually find that you can achieve a little more each day.

Emotional adjustment

All surgery is accompanied by emotions and this is particularly so with a caesarean. Relief, anger, resentment, disappointment and guilt are commonly experienced. Some new mothers may wish they had had a more active part in their delivery experiences, or that the decision for delivery by caesarean had been made earlier. It's important to remember that all these feelings – whether positive or positive – are entirely natural. If you are troubled in any way, you may find it helpful to discuss your feelings with the medical staff, who may be able to give you some information that will enhance your understanding and acceptance of your delivery experience.

The aim of this book

Caesarean Recovery will show you when and how to take the different steps toward your recovery, and it will guide you through the process in a safe and time-managed way. Don't put yourself under pressure by feeling that you have to rush things. Think of your recovery as a project that you can work through while you're getting to know your new baby.

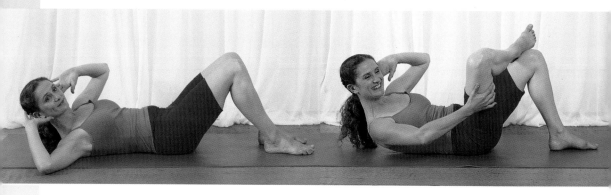

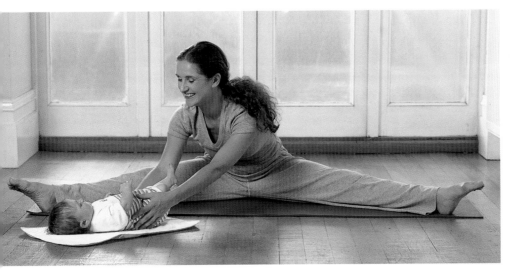

There are various movements that can be done at different stages, and these will assist you in moving up the mobility ladder. *Caesarean Recovery* will be your guide to the different stages, from your first attempts at sitting up in your hospital bed, through to standing independently, and then on to mastering your first exercises. When you are back at home with your new baby, *Caesarean Recovery* will then lead you through the next stage of mobility and strengthening, and provide a full exercise program to help you regain your fitness.

It is important to work carefully and safely. You will be advised when to begin each new set of exercises and how to build yourself back to full fitness. Not only this, but you also will have a chance to work on specific areas that are of concern after childbirth, such as the back, stomach and pelvic floor. Even after a caesarean delivery, it is possible to regain much of your previous abdominal strength – and get a trim stomach again. Finally, there are further suggestions on how to make time for your training, building your program gradually and continuing to benefit from it – right up until the next time you give birth.

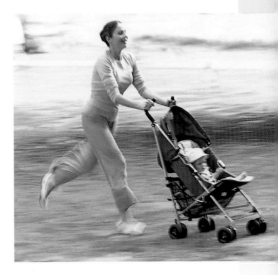

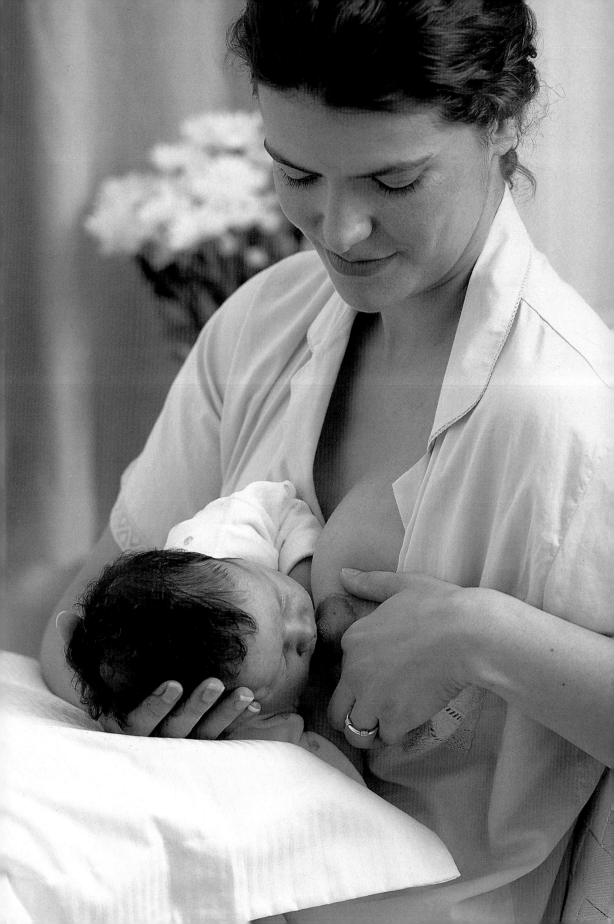

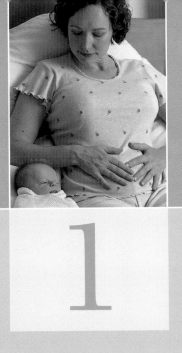

1

Having a caesarean

Whether your caesarean is planned or carried out as an emergency procedure, it's important to understand why it is being done. Knowing what will happen to you and your baby will make the whole experience less stressful. Although you are likely to feel a lot of discomfort in the days after the operation, it is really important that you get out of bed and start working on your mobility. Finding a comfortable breastfeeding position will help make nursing a pleasurable experience that will help you bond with your newborn.

Elective caesarean

An elective or planned caesarean section is decided upon and carried out before you actually go into labour. There are several reasons why you may be advised to have one, and it is important to understand why your doctor considers it necessary. Discuss all the implications so that you are fully prepared for the birth.

Reasons for an elective caesarean

The most common reason for an elective caesarean is a previous caesarean section. Many doctors are concerned that a vaginal birth after a caesarean (VBAC) may be too risky for a mother, particularly if the birth takes place in a small, local hospital. Mothers who have had a previous caesarean are often worried that the reason for the first caesarean may recur if they attempt a trial of labour and a vaginal delivery.

A planned caesarean may be suggested if you are carrying more than one baby, if your baby is considered to be too big to fit easily through your pelvis, or if he is lying in the wrong position in the uterus. Sometimes a baby or a mother has a physical anomaly or injury that may be made worse by a vaginal delivery or there is existing vaginal herpes infection, which could infect the baby if he was born vaginally.

If the mother or baby suffer from a serious medical condition, such as a heart problem, to avoid the stress of labour, a caesarean will be offered. Other reasons for an elective caesarean are if the mother has diabetes or eclampsia, a rare condition in which high blood pressure can lead to convulsions and, in extreme cases, even coma. Eclampsia is threatening to your health and to the well-being of your baby.

Twins
If the babies are in the wrong position for a vaginal birth a caesarean will be necessary.

Preparing yourself

Advance planning can help to make a caesarean a more satisfying experience. Choose childbirth classes that include information on

MAKING A BIRTH PLAN

Things you may want to include in your birth plan:

○ *I would like my partner to be present during the operation*

○ *I would like to be conscious*

○ *I want to be able to see my baby being born*

○ *I want to be able to touch my baby as soon as he is born*

○ *We would like to video or photograph the operation and my baby's birth*

○ *I want to hold my baby immediately after the birth*

○ *I would like to wait until the umbilical cord stops pulsating before it is clamped and cut*

○ *My partner would like to cut the cord*

○ *I want to breastfeed in the recovery room*

caesarean birth, and visit your hospital's labour and birth areas so that you are familiar with the type of room in which you will have your baby. Make a birth plan and then discuss your ideas with your doctor and midwife, who will be able to advise you about what is and isn't practical.

Make the delivery work for you

Ask your doctor if it is possible for you to wait until labour has begun before having the operation. Many experts believe that even a short time in labour will give a baby the advantages of uterine contractions – these stimulate the baby's breathing by squeezing out any fluid in the lungs and help to ensure maturity. If you are awake during the operation, don't be afraid to ask questions so that you understand what is happening.

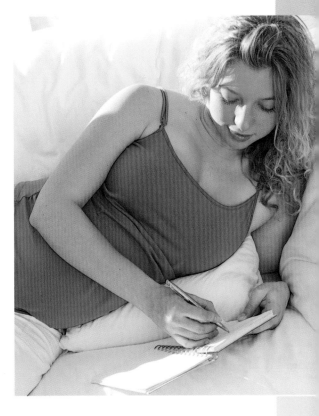

Unplanned or emergency caesarean

Occasionally it becomes obvious during labour that a caesarean is necessary, when you will be delivered more or less as a planned caesarean. A true emergency caesarean section (which will be more rushed) is carried out only when there is a serious complication. Even in an emergency situation, you and your birth partner should be given a brief explanation of why the operation is considered necessary.

Reasons for an unplanned caesarean

Once labour has begun a caesarean may be done if labour doesn't progress or progresses too slowly, as when the cervix stops dilating, or only dilates very slowly, or the baby does not move down into the pelvis – maybe because the mother's pelvis is too small or the baby is too big or his head is not in a good position. In such cases, both the mother and the baby can become too exhausted to proceed with a vaginal birth.

It may also be done if the baby's heartbeat shows he is not coping well with contractions (this is known as fetal distress) or if a mother develops moderae pregnancy-induced hypertension, or eclampsia during labour. A caesarean also will be needed if the baby is extremely premature or becomes at risk for trauma from the birth process.

Reasons for an emergency caesarean

If the placenta starts to become detached from the wall of the uterus (placental abruption) or labour causes a rupture to occur in the uterus, there is a risk of serious haemorrhage. so that an immediate emergency cesarean is required, followed by repair of the uterus. One will also be done if maternal medical conditions – pre-eclampsia or maternal heart disease worsen severely or there is a prolonged drop in the baby's heart rate. Other reasons may be excessive bleeding or if the baby's umbilical cord or a fetal part prolapses or protrudes through the cervix.

Placental abruption
The separation of the placenta from the uterus can lead to the formation of a pocket of blood, which necessitates urgent medical treatment.

If the caesarean is done as an emergency, the operation is much the same as a planned procedure save your partner will probably not be allowed in the operating theatre, you may have a general anaesthetic and a larger incision, and the process will be a lot more rushed.

A successful outcome

If there is any likelihood of your having an unplanned or emergency caesarean, try to ensure that the delivery is the best it can possibly be by adopting a positive outlook and cooperating fully with your healthcare team. Talk to your partner about the possibility of a caesarean so that you both understand what will happen if a caesarean becomes necessary. You also may find it useful to talk to other women who have been through the experience.

After you've had your baby, and before you leave hospital, ask your doctor or midwife to go through the reasons for the caesarean with you. Then, if in the future you decide to have another child, you will know whether you are likely to need another caesarean or not.

RISK FACTORS

There are some physical risks to the mother and baby in a caesarean birth.

For the mother:
* *Infection*
* *Increased bleeding*
* *Formation of blood clots*
* *Other post-surgical complications (such as adhesions)*
* *Longer recovery time after the birth*
* *With repeat caesareans, more scar tissue and damage to the bladder or bowel*

For the baby:
* *Breathing problems*
* *Low Apgar scores due to the anaesthesia*

Risks and benefits

Although caesareans are carried out regularly across the world, the procedure should not be undertaken lightly. As with any major surgery, there are risks such as haemorrhage, injury to other organs and infection associated with the operation. If you have more than two caesareans, there is an increased risk of placenta accreta (the placenta abnormally implants into the uterus), more scar tissue and greater chances of bleeding.

Before reaching a decision you and your doctor will have to weigh up any risks against the benefits. However, as most of the complications that result from a caesarean can be dealt with, the benefit of a speedy delivery will usually outweigh the risks to the mother and baby of remaining in labour when there are serious problems.

The procedure

Whether you have an elective or emergency cesarean, the operation is essentially the same. Your doctor should explain how the operation will be done and answer any questions you may have beforehand.

Before the operation

You will be asked not to eat or drink anything for at least eight hours before the operation (to prevent anaesthetic complications). You will probably be admitted to the hospital at least two hours before surgery. Your health and pregnancy history will be noted, a blood sample will then be taken, and you will be asked to provide a urine sample. Your blood pressure, pulse and temperature will be measured, and your doctor or midwife will listen to your baby's heartbeat. An intravenous infusion will be started to keep you hydrated. Before it is administered, an anaesthesiologist will discuss the type of pain relief – general or regional anaesthesia – that is to be used, (see page 20).

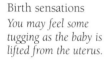

Birth sensations
You may feel some tugging as the baby is lifted from the uterus.

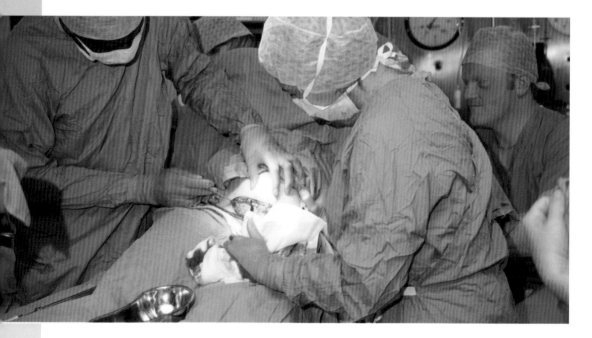

The caesarean section

Once the anaesthetic has taken effect, a bladder catheter will be inserted to drain urine, and your abdomen will be washed with antiseptic lotion. A small area of your lower abdomen will be shaved where the incision wll be made then your lower body will be covered with sterile drapes. The surgeon will then make a small incision into your abdomen (he or she should have discussed the type with you beforehand, see page 18). The most common is the "bikini cut" made horizontally just below the pubic hairline. A second incision will then be made through the lower section of the uterus. (The abdominal muscles aren't usually cut but are separated in the midline and pushed aside.) The surgeon then opens the amniotic sac and you may hear a whooshing sound as the fluid is sucked out. You will feel some movement and pressure as the surgeon reaches in and lifts out your baby. The placenta is then removed and the cord is clamped and cut. Once the baby is born and is breathing well, he will be brought to you and your partner to hold and enjoy while the surgeon sews up the incisions. The uterus is closed with stitches that dissolve in the body; the abdominal layers are stitched and finally the skin is sewn, taped or stapled together. The whole process takes about one hour.

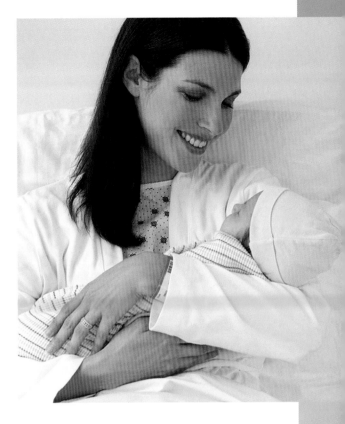

Getting acquainted
Once you are completely alert, your baby will be given to you so you can get to know each other.

After delivery

Once your incision is closed, you and your baby will be taken to a recovery room, where you will be monitored and you will be encouraged to breastfeed. Usually, you will spend between 1–4 hours in the recovery room before being taken to your room. The staff will keep a careful watch for the first 12–24 hours on your condition, and pain relief, which is important to speed recovery, also will be carefully monitored with medication being offered.

The incisions

During a caesarean two separate incisions are made – one through the skin and abdominal wall, and the other underneath this, through the uterine wall, to reach the amniotic sac and the baby. The cut that is visible on the outside is not necessarily in the same position as the internal incision into the uterus.

Surface incisions

Generally, a horizontal incision known as a bikini cut is made through the skin just above the pubic bone. The incision is just large enough for the baby to be taken out, and leaves a small, almost unnoticeable scar.

The classical cut

Rarely, in an emergency situation when the surgeon needs a large area in which to work or the baby must be removed quickly, a vertical incision called the classical cut is used. This incision extends from the navel down to the pubic area and allows more room for the baby's delivery so it helps to prevent birth trauma to both mother and baby. Birth trauma can occur if a baby is in a difficult position, there is more than one baby, or the lower part of the uterus isn't stretched enough to allow delivery through a transverse incision. The main drawbacks to this incision are a greater risk of blood loss during the operation, and a much higher chance of the uterus rupturing in subsequent labours. Having this incision means

Body beautiful
There is usually no reason why having a cesarean should prevent you from wearing a bikini in the future.

> **In the last eight years,
> I have had four caesareans...**
>
> Sophia *43 years*

I have had four children, all born by caesarean section. During the last operation my surgeon cut away all the old scar tissue so that now there is hardly any surface scarring left. Recently, I was asked to give a talk to my local prenatal group about what it was like to have had four cesareans. I think they expected me to be unhappy and disappointed at having had so many, and were surprised to find that I am not. I am just delighted with my healthy children.

that a woman will more likely need a caesarean for any subsequent pregnancies. The scar is also more unsightly. However, in an emergency situation, it is the quickest way of getting the baby out.

Uterine incisions

The most common cut is the low transverse incision, which runs from side to side across the lower part of the uterus. This is the part of the uterus that stretches rather than contracts, so there is more chance of the uterus healing to form a strong scar that will allow subsequent attempts at vaginal birth. One disadvantage of this type of incision is that it takes longer to perform, so it may not be possible if the caesarean is carried out as an emergency procedure.

When the classical cut is used, a similar vertical incision is then made through the uterine wall. There is also a low vertical incision that can be used if your baby is in an awkward position.

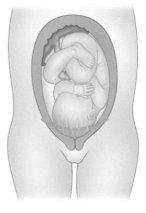

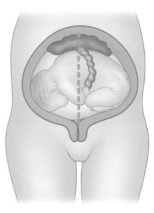

Uterine cuts
The low transverse incision (top) is most commonly used during a caesarean. The vertical incision (below) is used only in an emergency.

Anaesthesia

You will have a choice of pain relief during a caesarean. Regional methods anaesthetise only the abdominal area while general anaesthetics render you unconscious. Regional anaesthesia is more common but general anaesthesia works more quickly and may be given if a speedy delivery is necessary.

Regional anesthesia

In an elective caesarean you may be offered an epidural or a spinal block. Both of these options deaden any feeling in the lower half of the body but leave you awake and aware of what is happening. This means you can experience the birth of your baby without any pain and also can have your partner by your side for support and encouragement.

General anaesthesia

This is usually given in situations where regional anaesthesia is technically impossible or considered unsafe. You will breathe oxygen through a face mask for three to four minutes before medication is given through an intravenous drip. You should be asleep in 20–30 seconds. When you are unconscious, a tube will be inserted into your windpipe to help with your breathing and to

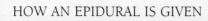

HOW AN EPIDURAL IS GIVEN

Anesthesia is injected into the space called the dura, just outside the outer membrane around the spinal cord. The drug is similar to that used by dentists and you will feel it like liquid ice numbing your belly, bottom and legs. Top-up injections, or a continuous drip of aanesthetic, are then given through a fine plastic tube that remains in place during the operation. An epidural takes about half an hour to set up and should provide complete pain relief.

prevent vomiting. When general anaesthesia is used, you will be constantly monitored by a specialist anaesthesiologist and your partner will not be allowed to stay with you for the delivery.

After surgery

You will be taken into a post-operative recovery room where you will remain for one to four hours, depending on the type of anesthesia you have had. If you've had an epidural or spinal block you will remain in the recovery room until feeling has returned to the lower half of your body and you are able to wriggle your legs. If you've had a general anaesthetic you will stay in the recovery room until you are fully alert.

Possible complications

The most common complication during spinal or epidural anaesthesia is a temporary drop in blood pressure. After a caesarean with regional anaesthesia, some women suffer severe headaches, while others complain of back pain.

A general anaesthetic may leave you feeling groggy, your throat may become dry and sore, and you may experience nausea and vomiting. If the anaesthetic contained morphine, you also may experience some itchiness all over your body. These side effects should disappear within 24–48 hours of the birth.

After an epidural
Your partner may be given your baby to hold while your incision is being stitched or stapled.

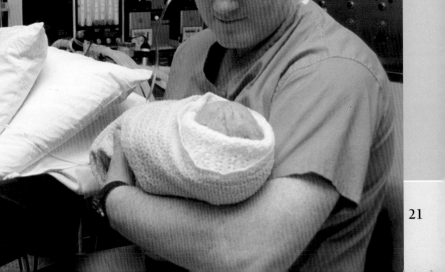

The first 24 hours

Along with any pain from your abdominal incision and any side effects from anaesthesia, you will now start to experience many of the same postpartum discomforts as a mother who has had a vaginal birth, such as uterine contractions, and lochia. Your doctor will be able to give you pain relief and can advise you how best to cope with any other problems you may be experiencing.

Pain relief

You are likely to begin to experience pain from the operation as the anaesthetic wears off, so it is important to find out what pain relief options are available to you. If you had an epidural or a spinal block, morphine analgesia can sometimes be given through the epidural catheter to help you through the first 24 hours.

A helping hand
Your nurse or midwife will help you to hold your baby in a comfortable position.

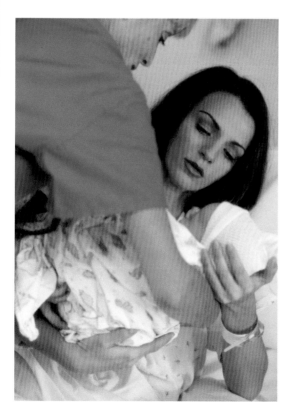

Alternatively, there may be a special pump on your intravenous (IV) line that allows you to dispense your own IV medications when it unlocks at preset times during the first 24-hour period. This is called patient-controlled analgesia (PCA). Or you may be offered intramuscular or oral drugs. The less pain you feel now, the easier you will find it to get up and start moving.

Feeding

If you are planning to breastfeed, you should start as soon as you feel able – in the recovery room, or perhaps an hour or two after surgery. Any pain relief medication that you are given will have been checked to make sure it's suitable for use with breastfeeding. You, yourself, may only be taking sips of water for the first 24 hours, but your IV will be keeping you hydrated.

Getting mobile

Although at this early stage you may not feel like getting out of bed, becoming mobile as quickly as possible is the best advice for post-caesarean mothers. The surgery and the anaesthesia can cause fluids to accumulate, which may lead to pneumonia, so movement is very important. Mobility improves lung function – as you breathe more deeply it boosts the circulation of blood, which lowers the risk of blood clots, improves digestion and helps the bowels start working again.

Within 6–8 hours, your carers will be there to help you to sit up, get you sitting on the side of the bed and start you walking short distances (see page 40). Bear in mind that you will need to get into a comfortable position every few hours to feed your baby anyway, so the sooner you can manage some degree of movement, the easier feeding will be.

Once you are up, use your hands, a pillow or a rolled-up towel placed against your abdomen to give you support. Most women will be encouraged to take a short walk every two hours. The pain of the operation may make you breathe rather shallowly, so deeper breathing will be encouraged as you walk. Deep breaths while lying down in bed are also a good idea (see page 39).

Walking
Although you may not feel like getting out of bed, walking will help to speed your recovery.

Other procedures

The bladder catheter that was inserted before your caesarean will usually be removed once you can walk to the bathroom. The IV line you had inserted before the operation will be kept in place until your intestines begin to work again. You will know this is happening when you start to experience rumbling in your stomach and gas pains. You can ease gas pain by avoiding carbonated drinks, or drinks that are very hot or very cold and by introducing bland, mild foods slowly. The more slowly you introduce solids the less gas and bloating you will experience (see also page 32).

Breastfeeding

Mothers successfully breastfeed their babies after having caesarean sections and go on to nurse them for as long as moms who have had vaginal deliveries. Studies show that it is the mother's commitment to breastfeeding that makes for success, rather than the ease of the delivery. If you are committed to the idea of breastfeeding then having a caesarean need not stop you.

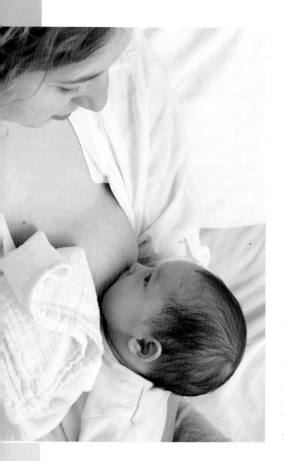

The first feed
You will be encouraged to put your baby to the breast as soon as possible after the birth.

Think positive!

Breastfeeding after a caesarean section may be an additional challenge for you at first, but this should not stop you doing it or detract from the pleasure you will get from nursing your baby.

Occasionally, hospitals have to separate a mother and baby after a caesarean – either because the baby needs special care, or because there have been complications with the mother. However, if there have been no complications, you can usually request that your baby remain with you so that you can start breastfeeding as soon after the birth as you like.

Advantages

Breastfeeding has many benefits for your baby, and these advantages apply when you've had a caesarean just as much as they do after a vaginal delivery. During the first few days your breasts produce colostrum, which, as well as being the ideal food for your baby, will give him important immunological advantages. Breastfeeding will also benefit you because your baby's sucking releases the hormone oxytocin, which encourages your uterus to contract. Breastfeeding within a couple of hours of the birth, when your baby's sucking urge is strongest, will be relatively pain-free because the anaesthetic will still be taking effect. This will help the bonding process between you

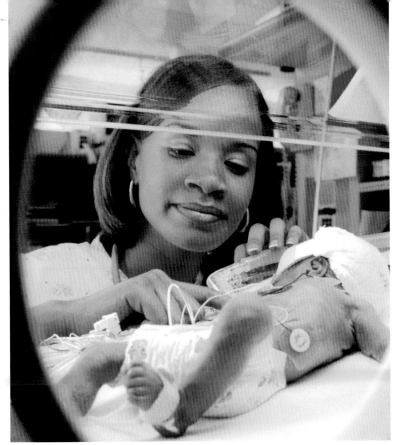

Special care
If the caesarean was as a result of complications during labour, your baby may need to spend some time being monitored in an incubator. However, during this time you will be encouraged to express milk so your baby can benefit from your milk's protective qualities.

and your baby before you start to feel any discomfort from the operation.

Obstacles to success

Babies born by caesarean can seem lethargic. This can be due to the mother's pain relief medication, but it may also be because the babies don't receive the same stimulation as when they are pushed down the birth canal. If your baby appears drowsy, he may need additional stimulation and encouragement to stay alert. This may also be true of you. If you've undergone a caesarean delivery under general anaesthetic you may be feeling really groggy and will need encouragement to attempt the first feed. Even after a regional anaesthesia, things can be slowed down and it is important to get your baby to feed as soon as possible, preferably within the first one to two hours. If this doesn't happen, a baby can quickly go into "down time" – a sleepy period that most newborns experience within hours of birth. Feeding your baby as soon as possible gives him nourishment before he gets too sleepy.

Early breastfeeding positions

There is no reason why you can't begin to breastfeed before the effects of the anaesthetic have worn off – in fact there are positive benefits to starting before you begin to feel tired and sore. If you have had regional anaesthesia, you may be able to feed your baby in the recovery room. After a general anaesthetic, you may need a bit longer to recover before you feel able to hold and feed your baby. Finding a comfortable position is the key to successful breastfeeding after a caesarean, so take your time and don't panic if things feel awkward at first.

FOOTBALL HOLD

For this position, you need to sit up straight, either in bed or, if you have been able to get out of bed, in a comfortable chair. Your scar will be protected by pillows, which will also support the weight of your baby.

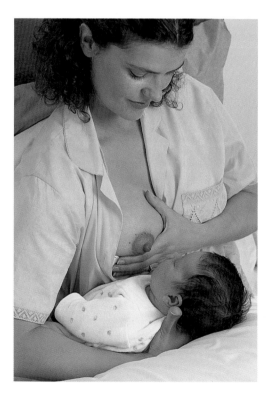

1 Sit in an upright position and put some pillows beside you, so that your baby is level with your nipple when you lay him down on them. With your baby facing toward you, hold him so that his body lies along the length of your inner forearm, with his bottom supported by the pillows and your hand supporting his neck and head. Make sure your baby's ears, shoulders and hips form a straight line. Draw your baby onto your breast, using your other hand to position your nipple in your baby's mouth.

2 Once your baby is latched on and sucking well, keep him close to your breast by wedging a pillow under the hand and wrist that are supporting him.

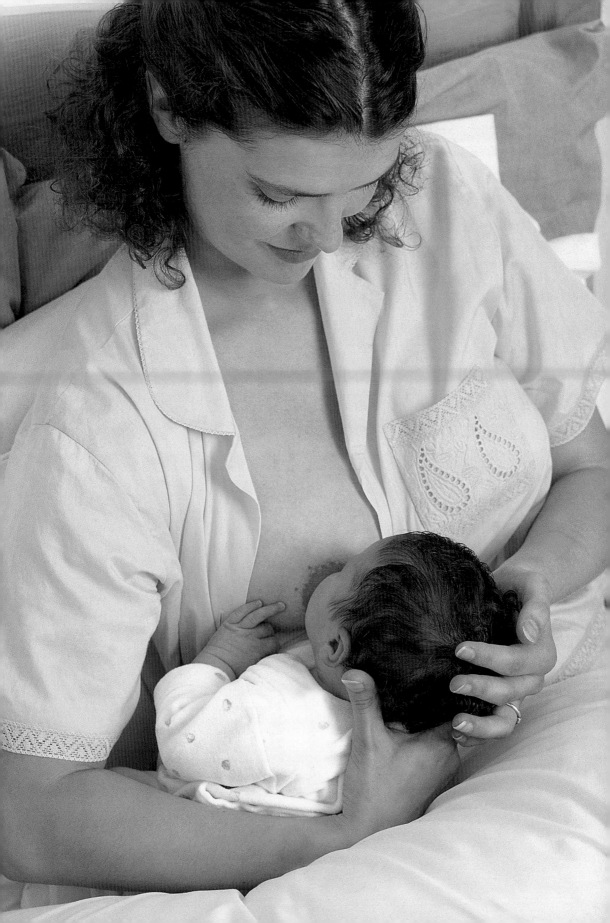

THE CROSS-CRADLE HOLD

For this position you need to sit up straight, either in bed or in a comfortable chair, holding your baby with the same arm as the football hold (see page 26), but this time you are going to breastfeed from the other breast.

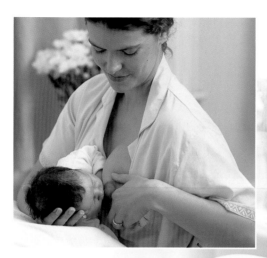

1 Put one or more pillows on your lap to bring your baby up to nipple level. Cradle him in your arm with the back of his neck in your hand rather than in the crook of your elbow. Turn your baby on his side so that he is facing you, with his nose in line with your nipple. Use your free hand to support your breast, and draw your baby toward you.

2 Once he is latched on and sucking well, you can place your free hand under his head to help support it.

LYING DOWN POSITION

You may find it is more comfortable to lie on your side in bed when you are trying to breastfeed. Some women find this position is uncomfortable if their scars are pulling – so do this only if it feels right for you.

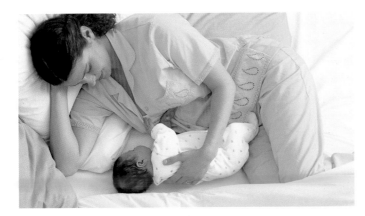

1 Lie on your side and ask someone to help you place pillows behind your back to keep you propped up. You may find it helps to have a pillow placed between your knees as well.

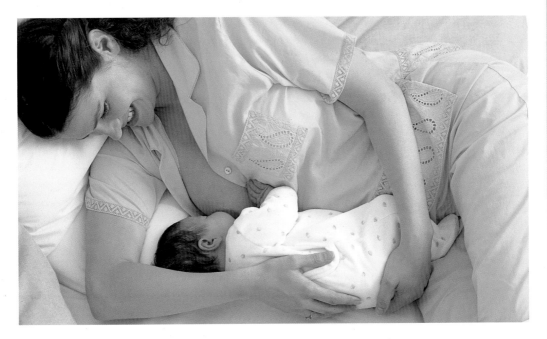

2 Place your baby on his side facing you, cradled in your arm, with his mouth lined up with your nipple. When he is ready, gently draw him onto your breast.

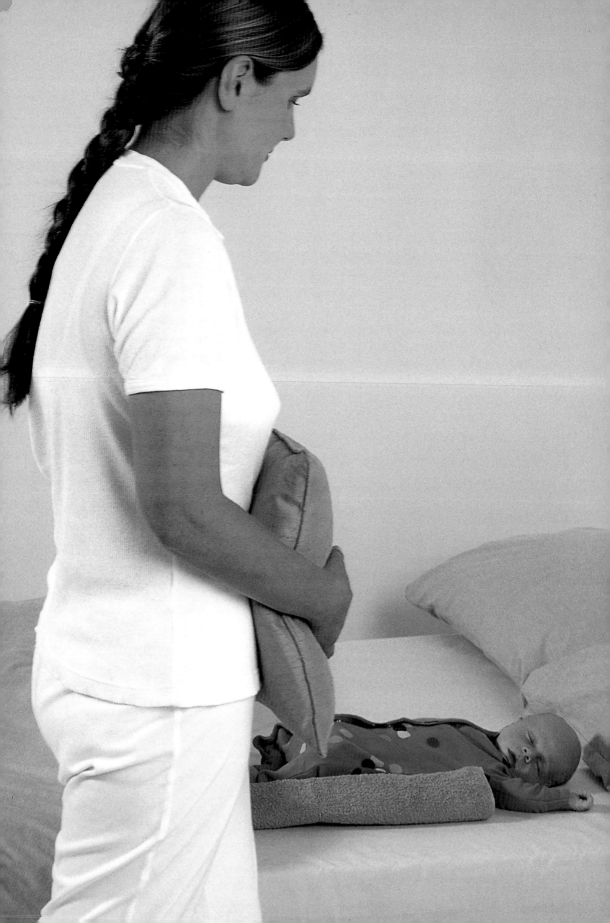

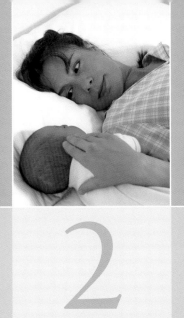

2

Week 1

This first post-operative week can be the most difficult because you are feeling sore and uncomfortable while looking after a demanding new baby. Your hormones may also be playing havoc with your emotions, leaving you weepy and tired. It's important to start your exercises as they will increase your mobility and make it easier for you when you go home. Before leaving the hospital, you need to make sure that everything is prepared for you and your baby, and that there will be plenty of support when you return home.

The first few days after surgery

After surgery, it can seem almost impossible to do the simplest tasks. Getting into certain positions can be difficult on your own, and even picking up your baby can feel painful. If you need help, ask for it. Although there will be some pain from the incision, you should not feel additional pain when nursing. If you make yourself comfortable, then you will feel more relaxed and so will your baby. Ultimately this will make for pleasant breastfeeding and a rewarding bonding time.

How to help yourself

Don't be afraid to experiment with different positions and to use cushions and pillows for support. Try to move a little more each day as the more mobile you are, the more quickly you will recover – so, even if it feels uncomfortable, persevere. You need to be sitting up and getting out of bed as much as you can, as soon as you can. It may not feel like the right thing to do, but it is – the more you move the easier moving will become.

Relieving the pain

Don't be a martyr to pain during these early days. Taking pain relief is not a sign of weakness – consider it an important aid to your recovery. If you are pain-free you will move around more freely and you will be able to hold and position your baby better. It's important that you don't wait for pain to become unbearable before you request pain medication. Your medical team cannot feel what you are feeling, so tell them before the pain builds. Pain relief taken in this way works much more effectively. If you have the pain under control, you will feel more motivated to persevere with breastfeeding.

GAS PAINS

These typically begin on the second or third day after delivery and improve once you are able to pass gas.

Things you can do that will help:
* *Get up and take short walks as often as possible, as soon after the birth as you can manage*
* *Change your position frequently when you are resting*
* *Rock gently backward and forward while sitting in a chair*
* *Wait for as long as you can before reintroducing solids into your diet*
* *Start with light meals that are easy to digest, such as toast, yogurt and soup*

Some women recommend the use of maternity belts during the first few weeks after a caesarean. These elastic supports for the stomach are mainly used during the last weeks of pregnancy. After your caesarean, try wrapping a maternity belt around your body and over your bandages – it will give you support and may give you some relief from discomfort. Before you use a maternity belt, check with your doctor or midwife that it is all right for you to do so.

Other discomforts

If you had a caesarean delivery after going through labour for hours, you may have perineal pain from pushing and from the number of internal exams you have had. Any discomfort in this area should disappear within a few days. It's possible that you may experience some pressure and discomfort when urinating for the first week or two after your delivery. Don't worry, this will gradually disappear as your body begins to heal. You should also be prepared for some itchiness around the incision as it heals.

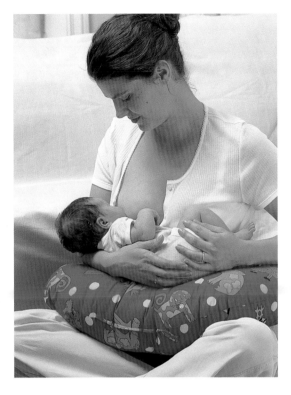

Comfort for you both
A specially designed pillow will make breastfeeding in the early days easier.

Succeeding with breastfeeding

You will need to be creative when it comes to breastfeeding positions (see page 26) and you may find that using a specially designed breastfeeding pillow will make you feel more comfortable when you are nursing your baby. These are designed to help put your baby in the correct position for breastfeeding while taking the pressure off the incision area.

If you are having problems with breastfeeding, you may want to contact a breastfeeding support group. Many of these have counsellors who will be able to help you with any problems you may encounter with breastfeeding. They will also be able to put you in touch with other caesarean mothers who can pass on helpful tips and advice.

Moods and depression

After giving birth many women experience a period of weepiness, known as the "baby blues." This tends to occur between the third and tenth day. For some, these emotions can become persistent, leading to feelings of inadequacy, panic and real fear. At this stage some women are diagnosed with postnatal depression.

Baby blues

Around half of new mothers suffer from the baby blues – feeling weepy for no reason, vague sadness, disappointment and emotional discontent. Such mothers become overly concerned with worries both small and large.

There may be other issues too, but usually with the baby blues, if a woman has good family support, these feelings recede naturally. Lack of sleep can be a big contributing factor; physical fatigue can reduce the amount of stress you can handle. Make sure you get sufficient rest, particularly when your baby is sleeping, and don't hesitate to take advantage of any help that is offered.

Postnatal depression

For about one in ten women these symptoms do not go away, and in fact worsen. Sometimes depressive symptoms kick in a few weeks or even months after the birth. Postnatal depression can be severe and have far-reaching effects, so it needs to be treated as quickly as possible.

Caesarean trauma

With the prevalence of caesarean births has come a greater awareness of the psychological aspects of the procedure.

SYMPTOMS TO LOOK OUT FOR

If virtually all of these negative feelings occur and they persist for any length of time you should seek medical help.

* *Worry about breastfeeding*
* *Getting angry at a friend who hasn't called*
* *Anxiety about how your partner feels toward you*
* *Fears about your baby's health*
* *Excessive crying*
* *Lethargy and sleeping problems*
* *Panic attacks*
* *Irritability and forgetfulness*
* *Feelings of being overwhelmed*
* *Feelings of hate toward your baby and/or your partner*
* *Low self-esteem*
* *Loss of libido*

Many healthcare providers now acknowledge that having a caesarean is not only a major surgical intervention, but also an emotional experience that can have powerful psychological effects on a woman's ability to adapt to motherhood. A woman's perception of her birth experience after a aesarean can be influenced by many factors: her values and beliefs, her expectations, the reason for her caesarean and her health afterward. Some women do not recover as well as others from the physical or mental trauma of a difficult birth.

Caesarean birth ranks up there with difficult life experiences, and it can leave its mark. Studies have shown that women who experienced emergency caesareans – with their obvious lack of control for the mother – can develop feelings of low self-esteem, disappointment and failure, whereas women who share in the decision making and are fully informed, experience a greater sense of satisfaction with their birth experiences.

Irritable baby
It can be hard to cope with an irritable baby when you are depressed, so ask for help.

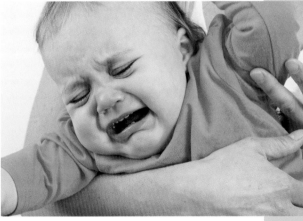

For some women the trauma of birth by caesarean – and other intrusive procedures – can be so great that they can suffer from post-traumatic stress disorder. PTSD is defined as a psychiatric disorder that develops from a perceived or actual threat of death or harm. There is also a severe mental illness known as puerperal psychosis with psychological symptoms that also can occur after childbirth. About 1 in 1,000 women suffer from this intense and dangerous form of depression, in which the mother can become out of touch with reality and feel manic, depressed or both. Puerperal psychosis usually requires hospital treatment, but most women make a full recovery in a matter of weeks.

Other causes

No single cause for the various types of postnatal depression has been precisely defined; rather, a variety of theories and factors have been put forward as contributors. These include:

* Having physical problems to recover from, or bad memories resurfacing from a childhood experience

* Hormonal changes at the end of a woman's pregnancy that affect her brain chemistry
* A baby who is irritable and sleeps hardly at all
* Lack of support from partner and family
* Being a perfectionist or suffering from low self-esteem
* Unhappiness over the labour and birth
* Previous postnatal depression

There are many other contributing factors that could be listed too, but the important issue is knowing how to address the problem once it has been identified.

Getting help

The first thing you should do is consult your own GP if you – or your partner – perceives there may be a problem with depression. Today, treatment for postnatal depression includes counselling in the form of groups or individual psychotherapy, and antidepressant medication. In rare cases hospitalisation may be required. Your doctor will also want to rule out any medical cause for your depression, such as thyroid disease.

If you feel uncomfortable about talking to your GP, or you are unsure whether you actually have depression, there are organisations that specialise in the condition. Usually the website will display a helpline number which you can use to talk to a counsellor.

If you feel able to discuss your feelings, talk to friends and family. Not only will this help you but also it will alert them to how you feel so that they can respond accordingly. Ask them for help so that you can relax for a while. Get your partner, a family member or a friend to look after the baby so you can have a good night's sleep.

Helping yourself

Try to do some exercise – this will release endorphins, which will help relieve tension and overcome frustrations. Try to get out of the house at least once a day, even if it's only for half an hour or so. Remember to drink plenty of fluids (water and orange juice mixed 50:50 is a good high-energy drink) and to eat regular, healthy meals. With help, these feelings of depression can be overcome, so never ignore the symptoms.

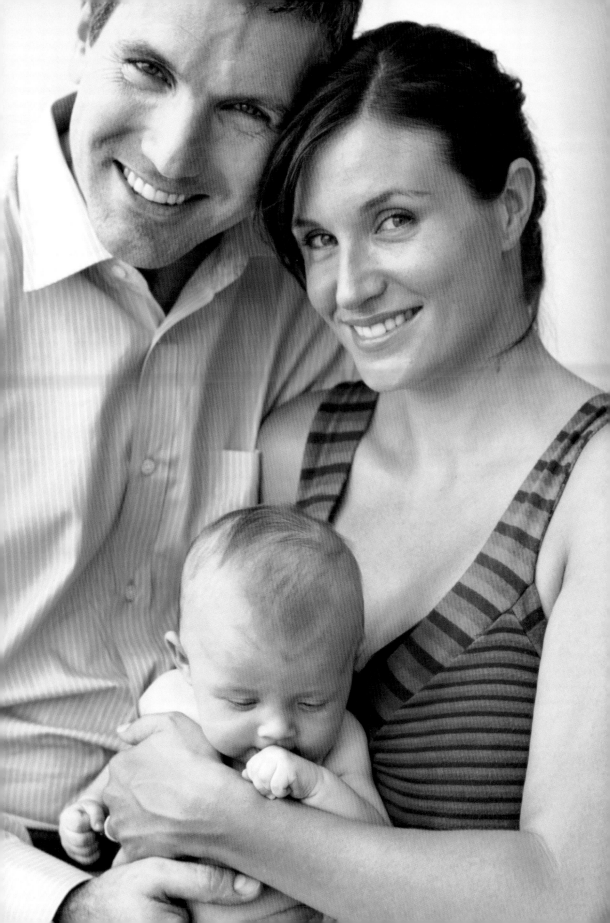

Days 1–4

While you are in hospital you will be busy recovering, and feeding and enjoying your new baby – but don't forget to put a few minutes a day aside for a short session of exercise. It may not be exercise in the way you would normally think of it, but even small movements will gradually strengthen your body and boost your circulation, so it is very important to do them.

Start by sitting, standing and walking, and then try the simple exercises below. Take it slowly and work your way through them. Remember that you will tire very easily, so don't be surprised if after only a few repetitions of a simple exercise you are fatigued. Rest at this point and try again later.

Feet circling and flexing

This will help to boost the circulation, particularly in your legs, and will help to prevent cramps.

Lying on your bed or sitting in a chair, start by relaxing completely, then circle your feet, one at a time. Think of drawing a large circle with your big toe, first in one direction and then in the other. Then flex each foot by pulling your toes back toward your shin, and then point your foot the other way so that you feel your calf muscle contract. Do both these exercises 2 or 3 times. Repeat twice in the day.

DEEP BREATHING

Breathing deeply helps you get rid of any lingering anaesthetic and will also help you get in touch with how your stomach area feels. Start with gentle breathing and gradually build up to deeper and deeper breaths.

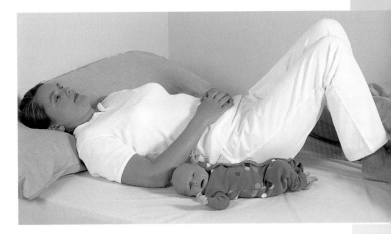

1 Lie on your back and bend your knees slightly. Place your hands on your upper chest and inhale. Try to aim the breath toward your hands then press your chest flatter as you expel the air.

2 Now take the breath a little further down your body. Place your hands over your ribs so that you can feel your lungs expanding as you breathe in. Then expel the air as before.

3 Try to push your breath even further down your body so that it reaches your stomach. This will stimulate the tissues around your scar. Support your incision by placing your hands gently over the area. Now take some deeper breaths in and out and feel the air reach your stomach. Repeat 3 or 4 times.

SITTING UP

This will feel very difficult to begin with, but remember that stretching and lengthening the muscles will ultimately help you feel more comfortable. Begin very slowly, and gradually ease yourself into each position.

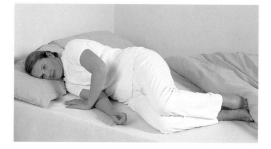 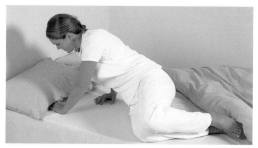

1 Bend your knees slightly and roll onto your side, bringing both knees with you.

2 Turn your head and use your hands to push yourself up into a seated position. As you make the initial push, the pull on your scar will feel really uncomfortable, but keep pushing with your arms until you are sitting up. Stay there for a few moments.

3 Now, start to take the weight onto your hands so that you can wiggle your hips back underneath you. Try to sit up as straight as possible. Take some deep breaths and start to lift up through your rib cage to straighten your spine. Try to relax your shoulders and let them fall downward as you lift up. Keep this lift and breathing going for 5 breaths and then relax.

GETTING OUT OF BED

Once you can sit up, the next step is getting out of bed so that you are in an upright position. The sooner you can stand, the sooner you will be able to start walking again.

1 Bring yourself to sitting position (see left). Now move your legs slowly to the side of the bed. Use your hands to push yourself forward and ease your feet down to the floor. Now push yourself up to a standing position. You will be crouched over at first.

2 Press a pillow or cushion firmly against your scar until it feels supported. As you do this, try to lift your upper body. Now try to straighten your torso, and then straighten your legs. You may need to try this several times before you succeed. Each time, try to come up to a straighter position.

Walking

Once you feel more comfortable on your feet you can start to take some small steps.

Keeping a pillow or cushion pressed against your scar, walk slowly ahead. As you walk, try to keep your head up. Breathe in through your mouth and out again. Keep going for several minutes before you return to your bed.

The pelvic floor muscles are the ones that you use when you want to urinate or defecate, and are the muscles you would have used to push your baby out if you'd had a vaginal birth. They will have been stretched and weakened during pregnancy. It is important to strengthen these muscles. You can do this by contracting the area around your vagina and anus. Hold it for 30 seconds. Do 8 contractions each time.

Stand and reach up

Try to stand tall at least twice each day, as this will get your muscles and joints moving.

Sitting on the edge of the bed, lever yourself onto your feet and come up to a standing position. Stay like this for a couple of seconds to get your balance and adjust to the feeling of discomfort around your incision. Now stand up as straight as you can. Think about contracting your back muscles to widen and stretch your chest. Try to lift up from your waist, slowly pulling away from your natural reaction to hunch over. If the position is too uncomfortable relax forward for a minute and try again.

Coughing

Hospitals recommend gentle coughing to stimulate the area around the stitches. This stimulation will promote healing around the wound. Do this several times a day.

Bring yourself into a sitting position (see page 40) and use your hands (or a pillow) to support your incision. Now try to cough 2 or 3 times, and then rest.

STOMACH PULL-INS

In these early days you may well find these pull-ins hard, as any feeling in this area will be limited. Although the lower layers of the incision will be healing fast, there will be a numbness around the area of the scar itself.

1 Lie down on the bed and contract your pelvic floor muscles (see opposite), then try to pull in your abdominals.

2 If you find it hard to know whether you are contracting your abdominal muscles, gently place both hands over your scar and concentrate on trying to pull your stomach away from your hands. Do 5 pull-ins and then rest. Do this twice a day.

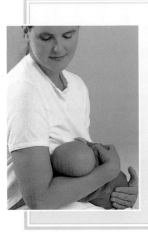

WHILE BREASTFEEDING

As you breastfeed, a hormone called oxytocin is released. It makes your uterus contract, so take advantage of this and pull in your stomach while you feed. Simply contract your stomach muscles for several seconds and then release. You may feel some discomfort at the sides of your scar as the uterus contracts. If it feels comfortable, aim to do 5–10 contractions each time you breastfeed. However, if it is very uncomfortable, leave the stomach pull-ins until later.

Days 4–7

As the days progress in hospital you should begin to feel more comfortable. You will still be tired after the operation and from the demands of your new baby, which, no doubt, will include being woken through the night. Remember, too, that having lots of visitors can be tiring, so be strict – or get your partner to be strict – and make sure you have plenty of time to rest. When you feel up to it, take 5 minutes to add some more exercises to your routine.

Go at your own pace

You will now be sitting up and getting out of bed each day. Although walking is still likely to be uncomfortable and tiring, you will find that you can go a little farther each time you get up. Try to stand up as straight as you can while you walk. Again, this will become easier as the days go by.

Although you will be spending a lot of time caring for your new baby, it is important to remember to find time for yourself, too. You should make the most of these few days in hospital and try to get as much rest as you can, while you can.

The exercises on the next pages follow on from what you have already achieved. They are very gentle, but you should still only do as many repetitions as feels comfortable. If 8 repetitions are recommended, and you only feel capable of doing 5, that's fine. Don't, at this stage, push yourself beyond what feels natural. Everyone is different and everyone recovers at a different rate, so the rule from here on is to use this book as a guide and listen to your body.

Your stay in hospital
Be sure to ask for advice if you or your partner have any concerns.

Pelvic tilts

This is a very important exercise as it is the key movement for realigning the spine. You should do this several times a day.

Contract your abdominals and press your lower back in to the bed. If you are able to do this correctly your pelvis will tilt. Do 4–8 pelvic tilts, holding each one for 2 seconds.

Leg slides

This exercise will strengthen your abdominals. At first, you may find that you cannot slide your legs very far.

Lie on your back with your knees bent and breathe normally. Now slide one foot down the bed, pushing the heel into the bed. As you extend your leg you are using your abdominals, so you may feel a slight twinge around your incision. Do 4 pushes with one heel and then change to the other leg. Rest between sets if you need to. Do this exercise every day.

HIP HITCHES

This exercise engages the side abdominal muscles – the external and internal oblique muscles. Each time you hitch your hips you are contracting your obliques and gently working them.

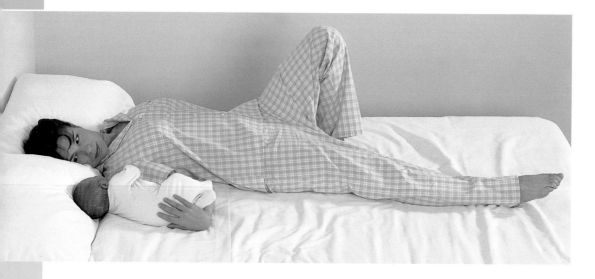

1 Lie on the bed or floor. Bend one knee up and stretch your other leg out, pointing your toes.

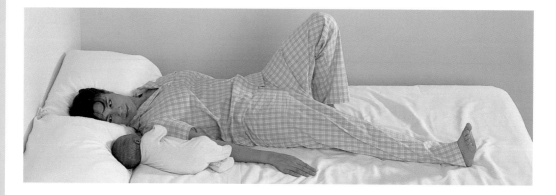

2 Pull the hip on the side of the bent leg up toward your shoulder, then release it. As you release, push your straight leg away from you. Change sides and repeat. Do 6–8 repetitions on each side. Try to do this twice a day.

KNEE ROLLS

You will feel your stomach working as you do this exercise. The twisting movement may pull on your scar, so only take your knees over as far as you can without feeling any discomfort.

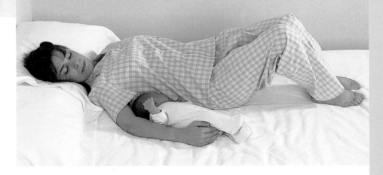

1 Lie on the bed or floor with both knees bent, and press your knees together. Put your hands out to the side for balance.

2 Now gently rock your knees to one side. Take your knees over so that your torso starts to twist. If you feel able, you can take your knees all the way to the bed. Do 3 knee sways to each side. Finish by straightening your legs and lying flat and relaxing for a few moments.

safety first

You should always be careful during the early days of your healing when getting into a sitting or standing position. When you are lying down, do not reach for something above your head, which makes you pull across diagonally, as this motion will put a strain on your scar. Always use both hands to push yourself up to an upright position.

BRIDGES

This move will use your abdominal muscles and work your buttock muscles as well. You may only be able to lift your hips a little way off the floor at first, but as your recovery progresses you will find that you can lift a little further each day.

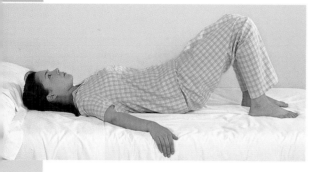

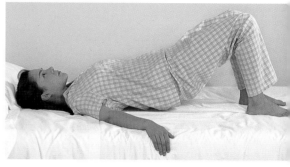

1 Lie flat on the bed with your knees bent. Place your arms out to the sides to help you balance.

2 Press your feet down and lift your hips slowly off the bed. Aim to peel your hips off the bed. Feel your coccyx lift, followed by the next sections of your spine until your hips lift into the air. Try to do 5 hip bridges every day.

ALL FOURS

This position may be uncomfortable to begin with – you may feel it is pulling slightly on your scar. If you can, stay in the basic all-fours position until it feels a little easier. Aim to keep your back flat, like a table, and breathe gently.

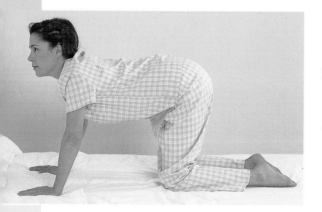

1 Get yourself slowly onto your hands and knees on the bed or the floor. Adjust your weight so that it is evenly spread over both your hands and knees. Once you can maintain the all-fours position without any discomfort, you can try to add some movement to this sequence.

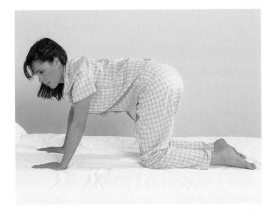 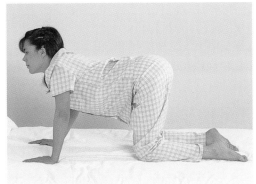

2 Press your hands and knees into the bed and try to achieve a similar move to the hip hitch (see page 46). Contract the side of your stomach (the oblique abdominals) so that you bring your hip up toward your shoulder. Repeat on the other side. If you are doing this move correctly you will feel as though you are wagging your tail. Do this move 5 times on each side.

3 While you are on all fours you can also try to press the middle of your back toward the floor. As you arch down you should feel your stomach stretching. Then, as you lift up to a straight, flat back again, concentrate on pulling in on your abdominals.

Variation

Finally, once the previous moves are easy for you, arch your back upward and then arch it down.

Ready to leave hospital

Most women usually spend a few days in hospital after a caesarean. However, if there have been any complications, you may need to stay in for longer. Hopefully, by the time you are ready to leave the hospital, you will be feeling a lot better than you did on day two.

How you may feel

You will be surprised by how differently you feel now from the way you felt in the first twenty-four hours. The pain you experienced early on will have become a lot milder, and you will find that you are starting to feel stronger. The important thing now is to take things slowly.

Physically

Your scar, by now, should be feeling less tender. If you are still in pain, keep taking pain relief to keep it under control and allow you to keep moving. Your sutures or stitches will be removed, leaving you with a scar. This may consist of quite a hard ridge along the incision, but it will gradually soften as it heals. The area may feel quite numb, which is natural, but the numbness will reduce as healing continues. You may, however, be left with some numbness directly around the scar for a long time. Some women never get all the feeling back in the area around their scars.

Hopefully you will have been mobile during your time in hospital and will be getting more confident about moving around – even with some discomfort. Keep doing all the exercises mentioned in the previous pages right up until you leave hospital.

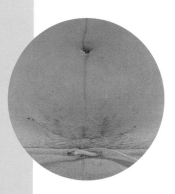

Know your scar
It is important that you become familiar with your scar so that you will know if any complications occur.

Mentally

Although you will no doubt be thrilled with your new baby, you are still having to cope with a lot of new demands at a time when you are recovering from a major operation, as well as the tiredness that comes from broken nights. Don't be surprised if you sometimes become weepy or feel rather down. It is quite natural to feel like this during this postpartum period.

> **" I just wanted to lie there and feel sorry for myself "**
>
> Sammy 26 years
>
> *I found it ironic that I was given so much attention during the late stages of my pregnancy compared to after the birth. I know this was due to the fact that I had pre-eclampsia, but I actually felt fine when I was expecting. Once I had the baby, the midwives' attitude seemed entirely different. They made me sit up, move about and do things for myself at a time when I just wanted to lie there and do nothing but feel sorry for myself.*

Sometimes the reaction of the nursing staff after you have had a caesarean can be a little surprising, especially if you have had a lot of attention prior to the delivery. You may find your healthcare team take a "get on with it" attitude to post-caesarean mothers, which can seem rather brusque. Don't be upset by this, as they are only trying to prepare you for your return home, where you will have to be more independent.

Although most mothers are anxious to get home and get settled back into familiar surroundings, it is quite normal to feel a little nervous to begin with. A supportive family can make all the difference, so take advantage of any help that is available. Your doctor, midwife and health visitor are also there to support you, so never be afraid to discuss any problems you may have or to ask for suggestions in solving particular problems.

Leaving hospital
Although you will feel excited, you may also feel a little nervous about how you will cope.

Being at home

If your caesarean was planned, you will probably have had time to organise things at home before going into hospital. If, however, it was an unplanned or emergency operation, you may need to rethink your plans for your first few weeks at home. Whichever type of delivery you had, you will be tired and sore at first. It always takes time to settle into a routine with a new baby, and this can take even longer after a caesarean because you have the additional discomfort of an operation.

Make yourself a feeding corner

If your home is busy with other children and adults around, having an area where you have everything set up in the way you want it can provide a little oasis of calm in the middle of all the activity. Ask your partner to help you set this up as soon as you get home.

You will need a quiet place that is comfortable and draft-free, away from where the rest of the family sit and play. Take your baby here each time he needs feeding. In this way you, your baby and your family will get used to respecting and protecting this space. If you feed your baby in several rooms around the house, then it may be an idea to set up a special feeding area in each of them.

Things you will need

First of all find a suitable chair in which to sit and feed your baby. Some chairs may not be suitable for use after a caesarean. Make sure the one you choose has enough room

Sitting comfortably
Make sure that the chair you use to feed your baby is comfortable with plenty of room for pillows or cushions.

for your elbows, along with cushions or pillows, so that comfortable breastfeeding positions are not restricted in any way.

Get yourself lots of pillows or cushions to prop up your arms and back as you feed. Use pillows to support your baby and cover your lower abdomen if it is still tender. Use a footstool or chair to prop your feet up on. This will help you maintain a good seated posture.

Keep a shawl or jumper handy, as well as your baby's blanket, so that you can use them for warmth, or indeed privacy, if you have unexpected guests. You may also want to place a basket beside you containing a burp cloth, nappies and changing items, breast pads and nipple cream.

Try to position some appropriate lighting nearby so that you can dim or brighten the lights as your mood dictates. A remote control CD player is a nice idea, too. You could put on some soothing music for your baby as he starts to doze after the feed. Alternatively, some rousing, noisy music may help keep a sleepy baby awake long enough to finish feeding.

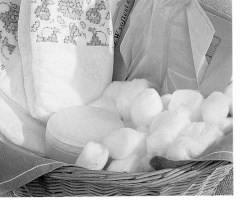

Changing basket
Have everything you need for your baby in one place so that you can change him easily.

Looking after yourself while feeding

You may also want to have within reach some nutritious snacks and fresh water in a sports bottle. You are likely to find that you become very thirsty when you are feeding, so it is important to keep up your fluid intake. Nutritious, non-perishable snacks such as nuts or dried fruit will maintain your blood-sugar levels.

A magazine or book to read may be a good idea, too. If your baby is a slow feeder you might grab some quality reading time as he feeds. You will find it useful to have a mobile phone near you, so that if the phone rings you won't need to get up if you want to answer it. If possible, avoid answering the phone when you are feeding – think of it as time for just you and the baby.

If you have other children, you might want to keep some supplies for them nearby, so that you don't have to get up while feeding. These might include: toys, colouring crayons and books, puzzles or story books, and the remote control for the TV so that you can flick on their favorite DVD. A snack and a drinking cup

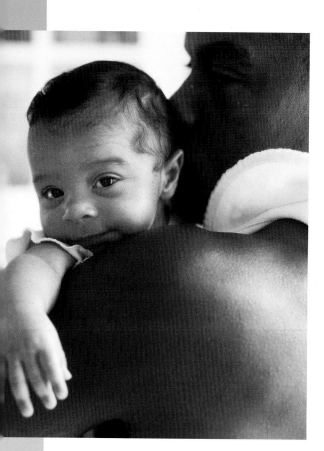

with a lid may also be a good idea – your toddler also might be glad of some refreshment. Another idea for keeping an older child amused is a photo album of his or her early years that you can look at together while you're feeding your child's new brother or sister.

Take it easy

There are some practical things you can do to help you through the first weeks after the birth which will also make you feel positive and in control. Most importantly, remember that you need rest. So try to sleep or at least relax when your baby sleeps, and accept all offers of help. If you don't get enough help, go ahead and ask for more. Family members or close friends usually jump at the chance of helping out in any way they can.

Although everyone will want to come and see you and your new baby, try to limit visitors in the first weeks so that you get plenty of rest as well as some peace and quiet. If you don't feel strong enough to explain to people that you don't feel up to seeing them, get your partner, a family member or a close friend to do it for you. No one will be offended if they know that you need your rest right now.

Get some rest
Encourage your partner to comfort your baby while you relax. It's a great bonding time for Dad and baby – and you'll also feel the benefit.

Be kind to yourself

Because you tire easily, you may also feel frustrated that everything you do seems to take so long. You need time to recover, so don't expect too much of yourself. Focus on one thing at a time and be prepared not to finish everything you want to get done – this way you won't become disappointed.

Relaxation techniques such as meditation or massage will help to relieve stress, and aromatherapy oils like lavender, marjoram, or camomile, added to a warm bath before you go to bed, will help you sleep. If you are breastfeeding, always check with a qualified practitioner to ensure that the oils you use are suitable.

When you are on your feet always try to stand as upright as possible. Do some exercises if you think of it, but if you don't, then don't worry. Instead, try to take some short walks – these will give you and your baby some fresh air and give you time to think about an exercise routine.

Eat small, regular, healthy snacks (see page 66) and drink plenty of water and juice so that you don't become dehydrated.

Don't rush things

Allow yourself plenty of time when dealing with your baby. Don't rush your daily routines, as they are an important part of your new relationship. You can postpone having to deal with others while you are busy with your baby by putting a message on your answering machine saying that you will try to get back to anyone who calls.

Expect to feel tired, overwhelmed at times and sore. You may even get some quite significant abdominal pains, especially while you are breastfeeding. All these things should settle down over the next few weeks.

Lying down practice

It is a good idea to do this after you have fed your baby, when your breasts are empty, as it will help you to get used to putting weight on your stomach again. Turn onto your hands and knees and walk your hands out, slowly lowering yourself down onto your stomach. Do this very slowly: thighs, abdomen, breasts, letting each part of the front of your body sink into the floor. Rest for a moment and get used to taking some weight on your stomach. Then, when you are ready, use your hands to push yourself back up onto your hands and knees again.

THINGS TO AVOID

Along with the practical things you can do to help yourself during this period there are some things that you should definitely avoid doing.

Don't:
* Lift anything heavier than your baby
* Drive for at least four weeks
* Rush to have to have sex. Wait until you feel comfortable, usually at around four to six weeks
* Worry about the state of your house
* Volunteer to cook for anyone but you and your family
* Overdo it. If you do, you will feel weepy and you may notice an increase in vaginal discharge (lochia)

Psychological adjustments

It may not be until you arrive home that the full impact of what you have been through really sinks in. After a caesarean, there are many issues that can concern a woman, and there are likely to be a number of questions that so far have been unanswered. Over time, some of these issues become more important than others.

Give yourself time to recover

You may experience feelings of inadequacy due to the fact that you are not as mobile, or feeling as energetic, as you would like. You may be frustrated because you can't move around easily, or pick things up – including your baby – in the spontaneous way you had imagined. This is natural and perfectly understandable. You have experienced a difficult birth and may not be getting the rest you need to recover, due to a wakeful and absorbing new baby. Added to this, you have an incision that needs care and may still be causing pain, and, if you were pushing before the caesarean was decided upon, you may even have perineal pain.

Broken nights
Lack of sleep makes things seem even more difficult, but try to focus on your beautiful newborn, and ask your partner to help.

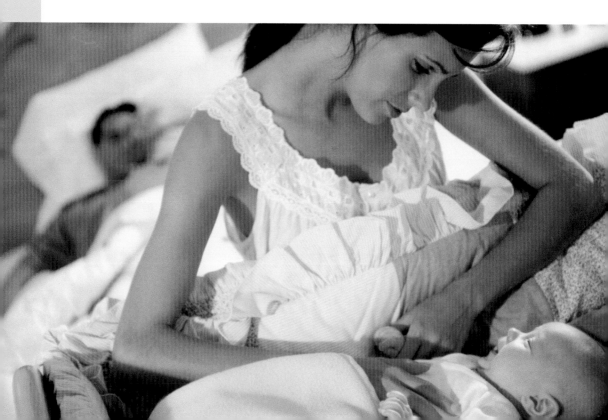

Some women report feeling dozy and "out of it" because of the drugs they have been given, and this can often affect their breastfeeding. Other women find breastfeeding hard because of the raised level of general discomfort. This is all natural – lack of sleep and pain make everything seem less rosy.

Feelings of resentment

You may experience feelings of anger or resentment when you look back at what happened at the birth. It may not have gone the way you had planned, or indeed dreamed about. If you attended birthing or prenatal classes and made a detailed birth plan, you may feel frustrated that it didn't go the way you wanted it to. Some women report feeling cheated that instead of pushing their babies out naturally, they were flat out on an operating table so that they barely saw their children entering the world. Others feel guilty, or think they are somehow less of a woman because they haven't managed a natural birth and had to have surgical intervention to deliver a baby. Again, these feelings are all natural and you shouldn't feel that you can't voice them. The important thing is to acknowledge them and discuss them with others. Your healthcare team will be able to help you if your feelings become overwhelming. Try to think as positively as you can and focus on your new baby.

Take comfort in the fact that very few births go perfectly to plan, despite the best labour-support facilities or carefully prepared birth plan. Remember, too, that there is no correct way to do things and your birth experience was still unique and valid, whether it was "textbook" or not. Finally, try to think of the scar as a positive thing too. These days the scar is likely to be below the knicker line, so you can still wear sexy underwear and bikinis without feeling self-conscious. Try to think of your scar as a battle wound that is testament to your commitment as a mother.

I did feel a little guilty that I hadn't had a "natural" birth. Although I had dreaded it, I still wanted to know what it felt like.

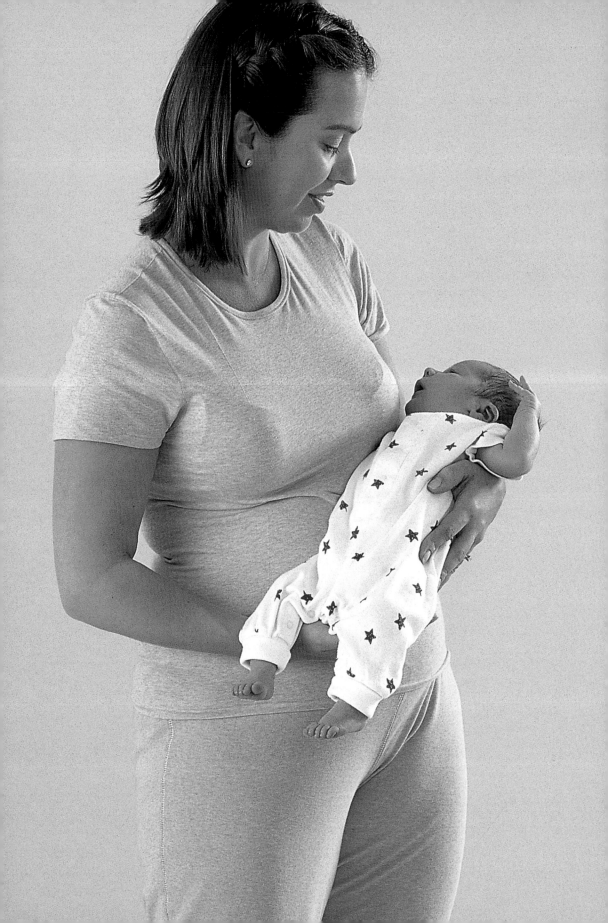

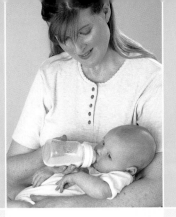

3

Weeks 2–12

Now you are home you will need to concentrate on getting your strength back. Eating healthily will play an important part in this recovery process and will also help you lose the extra weight you gained during pregnancy. You will need to look after your incision too, as the sooner this heals, the faster you will be able to get back to your pre-pregnancy state. Taking regular, gentle exercise will strengthen your muscles and help to give you the energy you will need as a new mum.

Caring for your incision

Although you will be busy looking after your new baby, and hopefully managing some exercises that will help with your mobility, you should also be taking time to look after your scar. Your scar should be healing well by now and shouldn't be causing you much discomfort.

How it looks and feels

There will be some pink, watery drainage from the incision at first, and you will have been shown how to clean the area and check for any redness or swelling. If the discharge continues for more than six weeks or if there is any inflammaton or pus-like fluid, you should tell your doctor or midwife right away, as you may have an infection.

Along the line of the incision, you may feel a hard ridge, which should gradually soften as time goes by. This area may also be numb and you may feel some tightening around the scar, or even deeper below the scar, as healing progresses. Sometimes this tightening is accompanied by a slight pulling sensation, deeper down, particularly round the two end points of the scar, when you move around or pick things up. Some women feel this tension around their scars for several years after the birth, but it should not be painful, merely a physical reminder. If you experience any discomfort, try placing a heated pad or a warm, moist towel against the area. Generally, if the scar is healing as it should, you will experience itching rather than pain; try not to scratch as this could cause infection. When your menstrual cycle has returned, you may find that the scar becomes tender around the time of your period.

Sometimes, if the scar tissue is rubbed or pinched, little blood blisters form on the incis-ion. These blisters appear black and may be

safety first

Although after the first 2–6 weeks there should only be minimal discomfort, don't try to lift anything heavy during this period (see page 69). Don't drive in the first four weeks either, because of the risk of haemorrhage if you have an accident. Only have sex when you are ready – this may not be for six weeks or more. Remind your partner that any position where the male is on top may be uncomfortable because of your scar and milk-filled breasts; try positions that keep his weight off you, such as a side-by-side position.

tender to touch, but usually disappear within a few days.

Practical tips

As soon as the bandage is off, you can wash the area with mild soap, rinse well and pat dry. You can shower or take a bath as usual, but always use mild, unscented soap when washing the incision site. After a bath or shower make sure the area is thoroughly dried and keep it dry by wearing loose clothing over the top during the day and leaving the area open at night.

If you are very overweight you will need to pay special attention to your scar. A lack of air to the incision site caused by overhanging rolls of skin can lead to infection, or the scar breaking down. Try to walk for exercise and stand straight when you are upright, as this will allow air to get to the area and promote healing.

Use pillows or cushions to support your body if you find it hard to get into a comfortable sleeping position. A cushion or pillow can also be used to protect the area when breastfeeding.

It is quite normal for a scar to take up to a year to heal completely. It will gradually fade as time goes by, but it is recommended that you keep it out of the sun for at least six months after the birth.

When to seek medical advice

If the bleeding from the incision stops and then starts again, or if it soaks more than one dressing every hour, or turns bright red, you should contact your doctor. However, if the area becomes painful, red, or swollen, or there is an unusual discharge, you must seek immediate medical attention.

NATURAL HEALING

There are a number of complementary therapies that may help soothe discomfort and promote healing.

○ ***Bach Flower remedies*** *Rescue Remedy and Star of Bethlehem may help to soothe the "shock" of the birth and make you feel more comfortable. Try taking a few drops in water several times a day.*

○ ***Arnica tincture*** *One drop taken in a glass of water every two hours may ease any bruising and swelling around the incision.*

○ ***Lavender oil*** *You can help your wound heal by adding 4 drops of lavender oil to warm, not hot, bath water. Mix well and then soak for 10 to 15 minutes twice a day.*

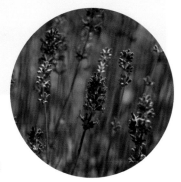

Healthy eating

Your goal is to eat and drink foods that will help you recover from your operation and, if you are breastfeeding, to produce sufficient milk for your baby. Some mothers become over-anxious about their diets after a caesarean, but there really is no need. It is much more important to relax and concentrate on getting better.

Ensuring a good milk supply

Rehydrate
Herbal and fruit teas make a refreshing and caffeine-free alternative to water or juice.

There are many old wives' tales that surround breastfeeding and it is wise to treat these with scepticism. Some unproved but popular recommendations include: that you must drink milk in order to produce it; that you shouldn't eat garlic and onions; that you must avoid spicy or curried foods and that you need to drink more than 12 glasses of water a day. In fact, studies show that a mother's diet has very little effect on the quality or composition of her breast milk.

While mothers in some areas of the world, for example Italy, regard garlic as something that might put babies off breast milk because it flavours it, mothers from other cultures – India, for example – think it actually helps successful feeding. The key is to keep your food intake varied and to make sure that you include plenty of fresh fruit and vegetables in your diet. This will keep your vitamin supply up and introduce your baby – via your milk – to a host of different tastes.

It is, however, recommended that you drink 6-10 250ml glasses a day of "approved" liquids, such as water, milk and juice. You may find that you experience an urge to drink as soon as you begin to breastfeed, so be guided by your body. Another way of gauging your fluid intake is to check your urine – if it is a pale golden colour you are drinking a sufficient amount, but if it is dark and pungent-smelling, you are dehydrated and should be drinking more.

If you are breastfeeding you will need an extra 450 to 550 calories each day. Some of these will come from fat stored during pregnancy, but the rest you will obtain from eating healthy meals and snacks.

Alcohol and caffeine

Alcohol passes from you to your baby in nearly the same concentration as when you drink it, so keep your intake to a minimum by drinking no more than one small glass of wine or beer a night. As caffeine can accumulate in your baby's system and may make him irritable and interfere with his sleeping, have no more than one cup of tea or coffee a day. Some soft drinks also contain caffeine, so check the label and don't imbibe more than 200mg per day.

If you're a vegetarian

You will need to pay special attention to your diet while breastfeeding to ensure that you obtain all the nutrients you need. As a nursing mother, your calcium requirement increases dramatically while breastfeeding, so if you don't eat dairy products – a main source of calcium – you will need to ensure that you eat plenty of potatoes, sweetcorn, dark leafy vegetables such as spinach, seeds, soy products and whole grain bread. You may also be advised to take vitamin B12 and calcium supplements.

Allergies

If there is a history of allergies in your family, you will probably have been told that breastfeeding your baby is especially important. Breast milk is the least allergenic and most digestible form of milk for your baby. If you do become aware, however, that something you eat seems to upset your baby, remove this food from your diet for a few days to see if there is

EXTRA DAILY NUTRIENTS FOR BREASTFEEDING MOTHERS

The percentage increase is based on the recommendations given for women who are not lactating.

Nutrient	Per day	% increase
Calories	500	26
Protein	11 g	24
Thiamin	0.2 mg	25
Riboflavin	0.5 mg	45
Niacin	2 mg	15
Vitamin B12	0.5 mg	33
Folate/folic acid	60 mcg	30
Vitamin C	30 mg	75
Vitamin A	350 mcg	58
Calcium	550 mg	80
Phosphorus	440 mg	80
Magnesium	50 mg	19
Zinc	6 mg	86
Copper	0.3 mg	25
Selenium	15 mcg	25

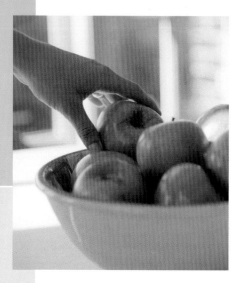

an improvement. It takes 4–6 hours after digestion for a food to have any effect on breast milk.

Foods thought to upset babies and possibly to cause colic include *brassicas* such as cabbage and broccoli, citrus fruit, grapes and chocolate. Very occasionally, if a baby shows symptoms of a milk-related disorder, a mother will be advised to avoid dairy products altogether during the period that she breastfeeds. If this is the case, you will be given specific dietary advice from your doctor.

Fruit for breakfast
Chopping some fresh fruit and adding it to cereal is an easy way to get extra vitamins into your diet.

Vitamin supplements

If you are already taking a pregnancy vitamin supplement you can continue with this while you breastfeed. An iron supplement may also be recommended – consult your doctor about this. These supplements also may be suggested if you are bottle feeding. If you are deficient in iron, include lots of dark green leafy vegetables in your diet. Drink a glass of orange juice – which contains vitamin C – with your meal to aid iron absorption from these vegetables. Additional calcium shouldn't be required if you include plenty of calcium-rich foods in your diet.

Food choices

The most important thing now is to eat well – include five portions of fruit and vegetables in your diet and eat three regular meals each day. Add to your plate of food, rather than take away a vegetable to every main meal and a piece of fruit to every breakfast or dinner.

You should also include plenty of dairy foods, oily fish, lean meat or vegetarian alternatives (see page 63), as well as lentils and beans, nuts and whole grain foods. If you snack, make sure that you do so healthily (see page 66) and avoid filling up on pastries, baked goods and candies.

Losing weight

Your body uses up calories more efficiently when you are breastfeeding. A breastfeeding mum potentially uses up 800 more calories a day than one who isn't breastfeeding – so if you stick to your normal eating pattern you should begin to lose weight safely and naturally.

MENU PLANNER FOR BREASTFEEDING MUMS

The following meal suggestions include all the essential vitamins and minerals required for breastfeeding. They are also delicious ideas – and good for you, too! Many are suitable for vegetarians.

Breakfast

Start your day with a fortified breakfast cereal that is enriched with folic acid and iron. Try adding fresh fruit, dried apricots and low-fat milk. Alternatively, eat a slice of whole-grain toast with your favourite spread. Eggs – boiled, poached or scrambled – on whole-wheat toast make a filling breakfast. Round your meal off with fruit juice or a smoothie.

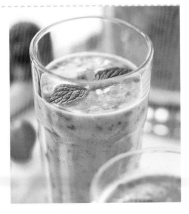

Lunch

A sandwich can be quick, delicious, filling and healthy. Try an open sandwich using different types of bread, such as ciabatta or focaccia, piled with your favourite toppings. Or make a pasta or couscous salad with chopped vegetables such as red or orange peppers. Accompany with a protein-rich food such as cold meat or sprinkle some chopped nuts in the salad. Finish off with fresh fruit salad.

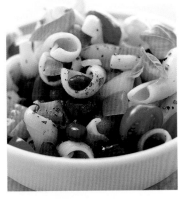

Dinner

Your main meal can be any dish containing meat, fish or other protein (lentils and beans), combined with a carbohydrate and vegetables. Try pan-fried chicken breast with broccoli and creamy mashed potato, grilled tuna with a baked potato and green salad or steamed tofu in spaghetti with sugar-snap peas and yellow peppers. Finish with a dessert to keep your energy levels up for feeding during the night. Try fruit with yogurt, meringue nests filled with apricots garnished with cream or rice pudding.

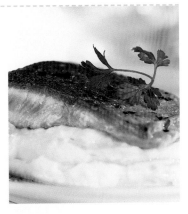

Whether you are breastfeeding or not, try not to focus on weight loss too much, in the first two months anyway, because you have so many other things to deal with during this time. In any event, don't be tempted to go on a crash diet or take weight-loss pills. They make it more difficult to lose weight in the long term and can make you even more tired.

If you put certain plans in place such as eating well and exercising gently (see page 72) then any extra weight will gradually come off. Bear in mind also that it will take you a full 10–14 months to get your strength, stamina and body-fat back to normal. Some women will do it faster, but this is a realistic target. Aiming for an unrealistic goal of "back in my shorts and jogging again" within six weeks will only put you under a lot of extra pressure and could lead to injury. After the first three months of breastfeeding, if you have naturally stopped losing weight, then reduce your calorie intake by 100 calories a day – your total daily intake should never be less than 1,800 calories – and begin to increase your activity level.

If you find you are losing too much weight, consult your doctor. It has been suggested that rapid weight loss can metabolise toxins from the body fat into the breast milk.

If you're not breastfeeding

Once you are up and about again, and you feel well recovered from your operation, you can start cutting back to your pre-pregnancy requirement of around 2,000 calories a day. But, even though you are not breastfeeding, it is important to eat healthily and to avoid crash dieting. You have had major surgery so you need to eat a healthy diet that gives you all the nutrients you need for your recovery.

NUTRIENT-PACKED SNACKS

To boost and vary your vitamin intake, try eating a few of these each day:

* *Nuts are great for boosting flagging energy – try cashew nuts for iron and almonds for calcium*
* *Pumpkin seeds and sunflower seeds supply you with protein and zinc*
* *Fresh fruit containing vitamin C will help iron absorption from other foods, and also supply phytonutrients*
* *Dried fruit such as figs, prunes and apricots are portable and delicious snacks that give you valuable amounts of iron, fibre and calcium*
* *Munch whole-wheat toast for energy, B vitamins, iron and some calcium*
* *Fortified breakfast cereals contain vitamins and minerals*
* *Yogurt and cheese are tasty calcium boosters*

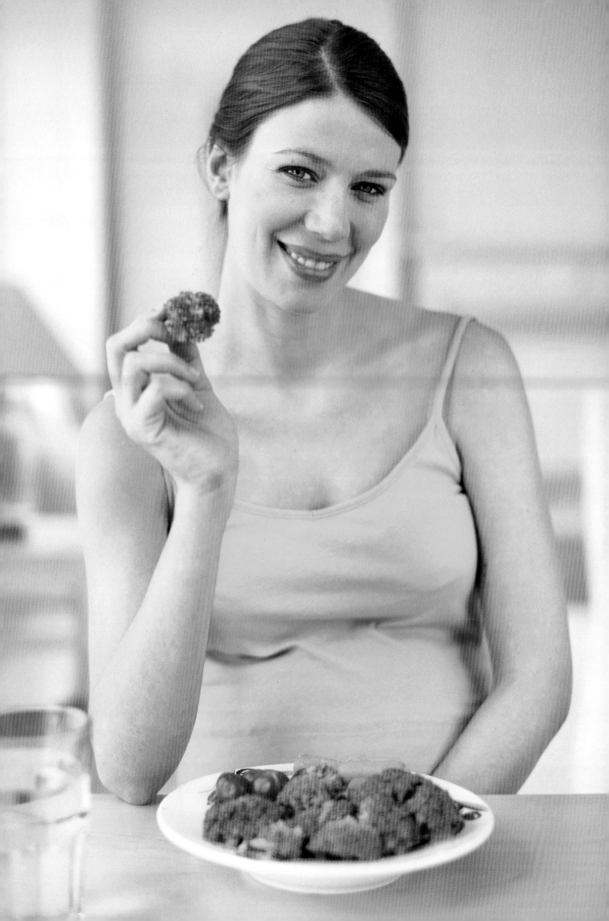

Weeks 2–6

Now you are back at home and a little more settled you can begin to do some regular exercise. Your baby probably won't have any kind of routine yet and neither, probably, will you. But don't let this put you off – you don't have to be completely organised to fit in a full fitness program. Think of exercise simply as a few moves you do each day – or every couple of days – that you fit in whenever and wherever you can. If you miss a couple of days it doesn't matter, so don't put pressure on yourself. Do what you can when you can, and remember that every little bit you do will help in the long term.

Overcoming the effects of relaxin

The hormone relaxin has been affecting your connective tissue throughout your pregnancy and if you are breastfeeding it is still present in your body. This hormone softens and loosens the cartilage, ligaments and tendons. Its purpose is to allow more movement in the fused joints of the pelvis to enable your baby to exit more easily. However, relaxin also affects your other joints, making areas such as your back and pelvis much less stable.

Sacroiliac joints

Prime areas for injury after giving birth are the sacroiliac joints, the points at which the pelvis joins the bottom of the spine, the sacrum. If you trace the bones of your hips with your fingers, up and over the curve at the side and follow the downward curve at the back, you will find two little hollows. These are your sacroiliac joints. Take note of this area and always treat it with respect.

Don't kick your legs out, and don't stand with all your weight on one leg for too long. When you bend down, do it slowly and, most important, be careful of your technique. If you follow the recommended techniques on the opposite page, not only will they protect your back and keep you injury-free, but they also will tone your stomach and major leg muscles, too.

HOW TO LIFT CORRECTLY

Many injuries are caused when new mums bend incorrectly. Injuries commonly occur when a mother leans over her baby, who is on the floor, to change his nappies or to pick him up, and then jumps up quickly, straining her joints in the process.

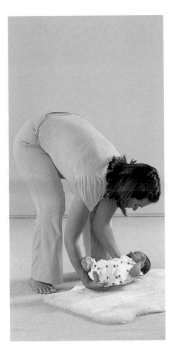

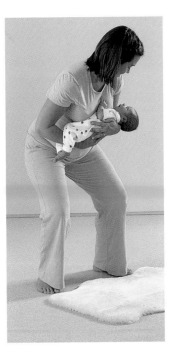

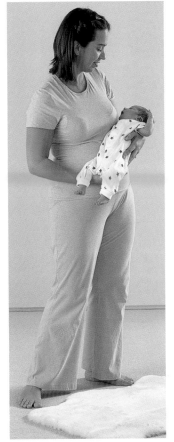

1 Stand as near as you can to your baby or to the object you wish to lift. Make sure your weight is equally distributed between both feet. Bend down into a squat position keeping your bottom pushed out behind you and your back in a straight line from shoulders to hips. Lean forward with the top of your body and arms and take hold of your baby (or the object).

2 Using your arm muscles to bring your baby close to you, begin gently to pick him up, simultaneously contracting your stomach and pelvic floor muscles.

3 Begin to straighten your upper body, pushing with your leg and buttock muscles until you have arrived at a full standing position.

You can have a trim stomach again

Once you have recovered from the trauma or drama of childbirth, one of the things you are most likely to be concerned with is your figure and whether you will ever get it back. The good news is that you can get your firm stomach back and you can begin work on this area properly from now on.

Although your stomach muscles may have been cut, they have also healed and therefore, with time and exercise, can be strong again. Your scar, however, is a different question. If you gain too much excess weight over the years, you will find that there is a tendency for some overhang to occur round your scar. So your aim now needs to be to keep your weight under control and your stomach as toned as possible.

Rectus diastasis

You also need to check that your abdominal muscles are intact before you start work on your stomach. *Rectus diastasis*, or separation, is a condition in which, instead of stretching over your baby as he grows, the rectus abdominal muscles in the front of your stomach pull away from the midline and separate. This can happen during pregnancy, so having a caesarean section doesn't prevent rectus diastasis from occurring.

Rectus diastasis only happens to some women and is not a major problem. It may occur as a result of the stomach muscles being too tight to stretch during pregnancy or because the muscles have been overexercised before pregnancy. However, what it does call for is a slightly different approach to stomach curls in the early weeks of your postnatal recovery program. If you have a gap – don't panic. This diastasis should naturally close as the weeks go on but you need to restore strength to your abdominal muscles. Follow the variation guidelines for rectus separation when performing the stomach exercises, as this will ensure you will not widen the gap with an incorrect technique.

safety first

The rectus separation techniques on the following pages can be used for many of the early stomach exercises. Although, in theory, the gap in the abdominals should go back together in the first few days, sometimes it can take longer. You can't physically perform an exercise to bring them back together, but you can certainly make sure your exercises are not making the separation any worse.

RECTUS DIASTASIS CHECK

Although your doctor should check for this before you leave hospital, just in case he or she hasn't or the condition has gone undiscovered, it's always a good idea to perform this self-test before starting any exercise program.

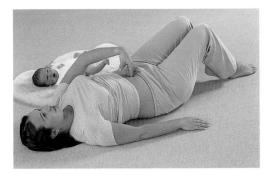

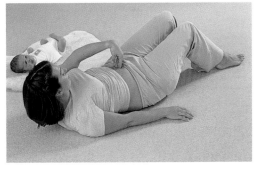

1 Lie on your back with your knees bent and feet flat on the floor. Take the middle three fingers of one hand and place them on your stomach horizontally, just below your tummy button.

2 Press in gently with your fingers and, at the same time, lift your head off the floor. As your head lifts, you should feel the muscles beneath your fingers react. If they repulse your fingers, there isn't a gap, but if they tighten around your fingers and feel soft and squidgy, the muscles have parted.

GOING UNDER COVER

During the course of a normal pregnancy, the most superficial of your abdominal muscles, the rectus abdominus, *which run down the middle of your stomach, become stretched. If they separate, however, and pull away from the midline (the central ligament or linea alba), this separation is known as diastasis. The gap may be the breadth of one finger or as much as two or three fingers. It's important when exercising to keep these muscles pulled together rather than increasing the gap.*

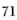

HEAD LIFTS

Curl-ups, which contract the abdominal muscles, are essential for getting your stomach back in shape. But you need to take things slowly. The first step toward proper curl-ups is the head lift.

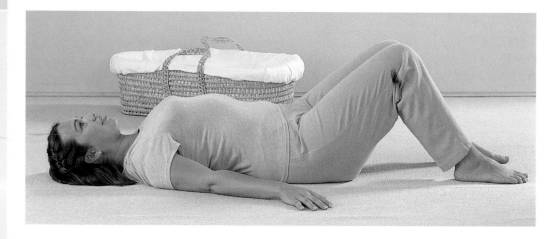

1 Wearing warm, non-restrictive clothes, lie on your back on the floor, with your knees bent and your feet flat on the floor. Place your hands down by your sides.

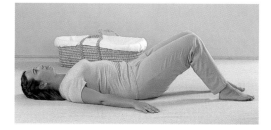

2 Start by performing the pelvic tilt, where you press your lower back against the floor and engage the pelvic and abdominal muscles.

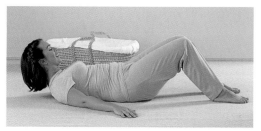

3 Now lift your head and focus on pulling in the stomach area. Look down the line of your body so that you can see and feel your muscles working. Hold this position for 2–3 seconds and release. When you lift your head you will feel your stomach muscles really contracting. Do as many of these head lifts as feels comfortable – up to 10 repetitions.

HEAD LIFTS WITH RECTUS SEPARATION

If you have got some degree of rectus separation, then forcing your way through a lot of sloppily performed sit-ups could make things worse. Take things slowly and build up gradually. Perform either of the following 8–10 times.

FINGER-GRIP TECHNIQUE

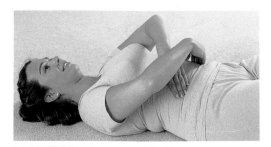 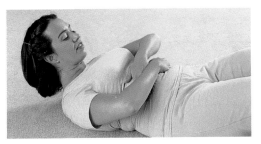

1 Lie on your back with your knees bent and your feet flat on the floor. Cross your arms so your hands fall on either side of your stomach. Gently press your lower back into the floor.

2 Perform the head lift as in step 3, opposite, but as you lift your head, use your fingers to pull the two sides of your stomach together. Slowly lower your head and release your finger grip on the way down.

SWEATSHIRT TECHNIQUE

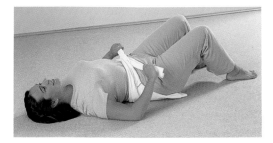 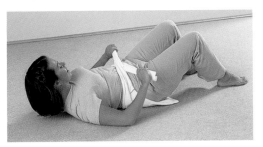

1 Another way to ensure that you are not widening the gap as you perform your head lift is to use a sweatshirt or other long-sleeved top. Wrap the top around your back with the two sleeves crossing over your midriff. Lie down on the floor and take hold of a sleeve with each hand.

2 Perform the head lift as in step 3, opposite, but as you lift, pull firmly on the sleeves so the shirt is pulled tightly across your middle. This will keep your muscles supported and together as you contract them. Release the squeeze as you lower your head to the floor.

KNEE TIPS

Similar to your first week's exercise, but this time you are going to allow your knees to fall completely over so that they rest on the floor. This will start to loosen up the waist as you twist, it will also start to stretch the muscles of your thighs a little.

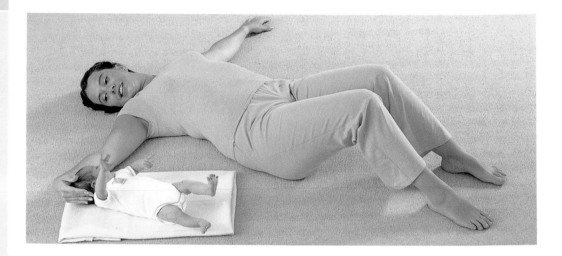

1 Lie on your back with knees bent and feet on the floor. Stretch out your arms along the floor, either side of your body.

2 Now gently tip your knees to one side, keeping your arms out to the side of you to aid your balance. You may feel a slight pulling across your lower abdomen and around your scar. If this happens, rest in this position for a few seconds to allow any discomfort to recede.

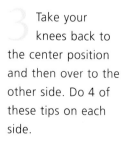

3 Take your knees back to the center position and then over to the other side. Do 4 of these tips on each side.

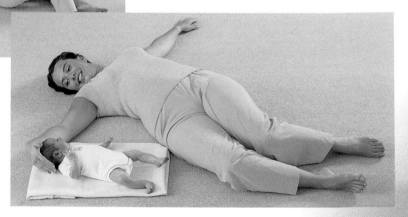

KNEE HUG-INS

This move will relax you and mobilise the front of your body. It will also give you a nice stretch across your lower back. If you can get your partner to press your knees in for you, it will feel even better.

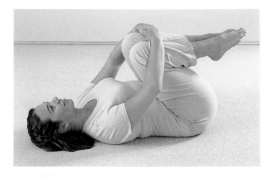 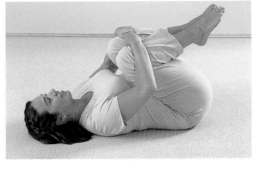

1 Lie on your back and bring both knees into your chest. Take hold of your knees with both hands. Inhale and exhale.

2 As you exhale, use your arms to pull your knees more fully into your chest. Repeat 8–10 times.

Under-knee variation

If you find it difficult to pull your knees into your chest, an easier version is to place your hands behind your knees and gently exert pressure with your hands to bring your knees closer to your head.

LEG CIRCLES

These will help to mobilise your hip joints and gently work the lower section of your abdominals. Keeping your lower back on the floor the whole time will give it a gentle massage, too.

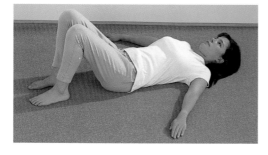

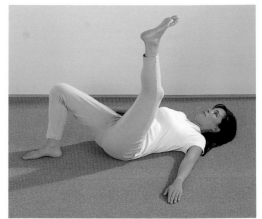

1 Lie on your back with your feet flat on the floor and take your arms out to the sides for balance.

2 Now raise one leg to the ceiling and slowly circle your foot in the air. Perform 8 large circles – first one way and then the other – change legs and repeat.

Variation
You can vary this move by lowering your leg slightly toward the floor and then taking it up again. Only go far enough to feel the abdominals tighten before lifting your leg again.

LEG LIFTS

Once you have mastered the leg circles on the opposite page you can progress to these leg lifts. This exercise will work your hip flexors (front of hip muscles) and will help to strengthen your abdominals.

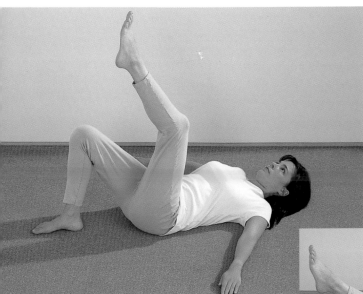

1 Lie on your back with one leg raised, in the same position as for leg circles. Try to straighten your leg completely and point your foot.

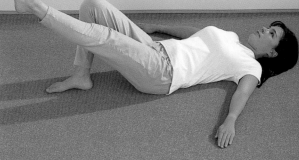

safety first

If you over-point your foot or over-strain your muscles while exercising, your muscles may cramp. If you experience cramp, stop exercising and press with both hands on the contracted muscle to help the muscle release. Then take hold of the area which is affected and stretch the muscle, gently rubbing the area with the flat of your hand to bring blood to the site.

2 With your leg extended and hands on the floor for support, lower your leg all the way to the floor. Do this slowly, aiming to keep your back flat on the floor as you bring your leg down. Rest your leg briefly on the floor and then raise it up again. Do 8 leg lifts on each side.

Weeks 7–12

As you continue to recover and feel stronger you can start to add more elements to your workout program. Always begin by using the exercises from the previous weeks as your warm-up moves, and then gradually add the following exercises. By the end of three months you should be able to do all these exercises with ease.

Be kind to yourself

If you have had a particularly wakeful night with the baby, you may not feel like doing 40 minutes of exercise. Do what you can manage – even if it's only five minutes. These five minutes, done regularly, will still make a difference, and once things have settled down you will be able to fit in a longer workout time.

Full cobra

This move will stretch out the front of your body and help exercise your lower spine. Don't worry if you feel the scar area being stretched slightly along with your abdominals.

Lie on your stomach and place your hands on the floor, underneath your shoulders. Now press back and straighten your arms so that your back arches. Hold this position for several seconds. Repeat 8 times.

Working your back

Exercises that help to strengthen your back are very important for your postnatal recovery. During your pregnancy your back was put under a lot of stress and strain, and your ligaments will have been softened by the hormone relaxin, so you are likely to have experienced some backache. You probably found it difficult to do any back work from the time you began to show. Your protruding stomach would have made it almost impossible because nearly all back work involves lying face down.

Now you should start to reintroduce some back-strengthening exercises. You may not feel you are achieving much at first because it takes time to get these muscles into shape again. But, by working on these exercises every day, you will soon notice a difference. You may find some of these exercises uncomfortable if you are breastfeeding and your breasts are full. Try to find the time to exercise after you have fed your baby, when your breasts are empty, as this will make it easier for you.

Full hyper-extensions

This move will work the muscles that line the spine – the *erector spinae* muscles. Don't worry if initially you cannot lift very far off the floor. As you get stronger, you will be able to lift your entire upper body – shoulders, chest and rib cage.

Lie flat on your front and cross your hands behind your back. Lift your head and shoulders off the floor as far as you can. Hold for a second and then release. Repeat 8 times.

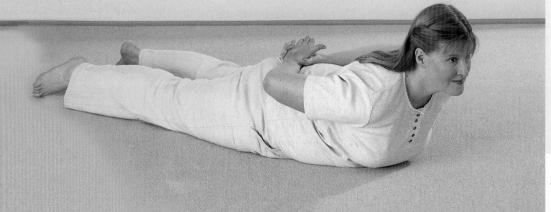

PELVIC TILT SERIES

This exercise makes use of the abdominals to remind your body of good alignment, and strengthens the whole torso in the process. As you extend a leg or change the arm position, you will feel the work getting harder.

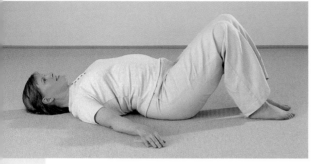

1 Lie on your back with both your knees bent and your feet on the floor. Place your hands by your sides and perform 8 pelvic tilts (see page 110). Don't forget that you need to pull in on the abdominals and press your lower back into the floor to effect a pelvic tilt.

2 Now extend one leg and point your toes. Leave your arms out to your sides to give you balance. Perform 8 more pelvic tilts. Now extend the other leg and, keeping your arms in the same position, perform another 8 pelvic tilts.

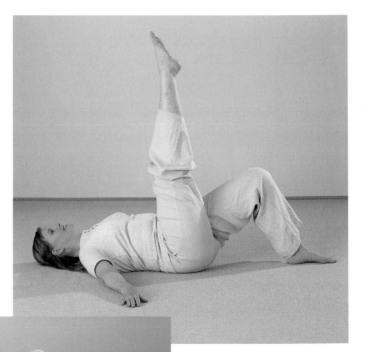

3 To finish up, bend your legs and take your arms up above your head to perform a final 8 pelvic tilts.

LAMBADA LILT

This sequence will help you get some mobility back in your torso and awaken your body's memory of lithe movement in this area. If your baby is awake, why not hold him while you do these movements?

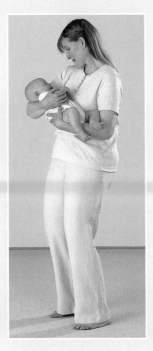 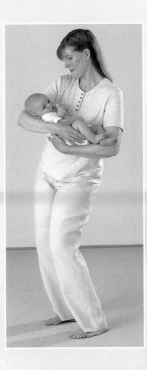

1 Stand with your feet hip width apart and perform a pelvic tilt. Over-emphasise the tilt and really tuck your hips under, then release your hips right to the back. Do this 4 times.

2 Now start to circle your hips, first one way then the other. Then try to draw a figure of 8 with your hips, in one direction, then the other.

3 Finally, try moving your rib cage one way and your hips the other. Keep going with this movement from side to side until it is a fluid and snaky like that of a Lambada dancer. Keep these moves going for 4–5 minutes.

HIGH KICKS

You are using and strengthening your abdominals with this move, as well as the hip flexor muscles that cross your hips and attach to your thighs. These muscles support the abdominals during leg movements.

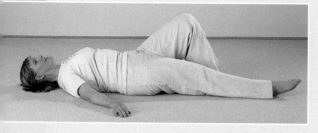

1 Lie on your back and place your hands by your sides. Bend one leg and straighten the other with a pointed toe, contracting your abdominals.

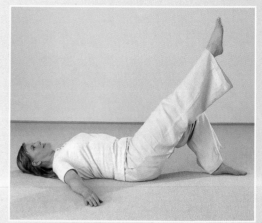

2 Lift your extended leg up into the air as high as you can and slowly lower it again. Do 8 lifts on each leg in this way.

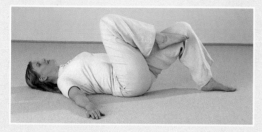

3 To alter the move, keep your arms out to your sides and bend your leg, bringing it into your chest.

4 Now extend your leg up to the ceiling and then lower it slowly back down to the floor, keeping it straight. Do a further 8 lifts on each leg in this way.

CURL-UPS

Now you are ready to perform full curl-ups. Be meticulous with each lift you do, checking that you have lifted your shoulder blades off the floor and that you are pulling in on your abdominals as well.

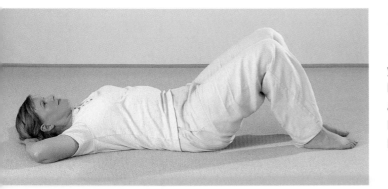

1 Lie on your back with your knees bent and your hands behind your head. Breathe in and then, as you breathe out, lift your head and shoulders up as high as you can.

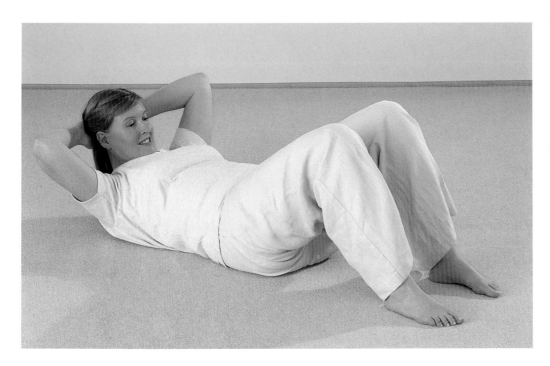

2 Look down along the line of your navel and hold this position for two seconds before lowering again. When you look along the line of your stomach, try to keep your abdominals from bulging out too much. Build up to performing 20 slow, controlled curls.

BASIC SQUAT

This is a great move for toning the bottom and thighs. It is also the move you use when lifting something (see page 69). Using it will prevent you from stooping over and making your back ache, and it will work your legs while you do it.

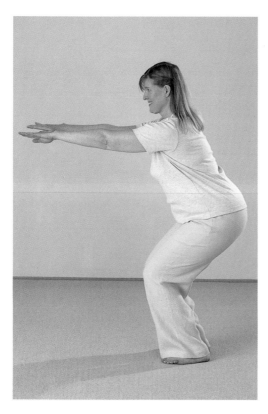 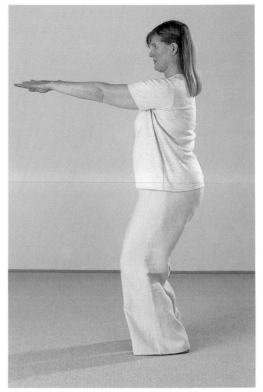

1 Stand with your feet hip-width apart with your weight on the balls of your feet. Tilt your pelvis, keeping your abdominals tight. Now, with your arms outstretched, push your backside out behind you as you bend your legs. You should feel the weight of your body over your heels.

2 Hold this position while you check your alignment. Your body should be straight from your hips up to your shoulders with your stomach pulled in. Now press through your legs and use your buttocks to push yourself up and bring you to standing. Perform this move 8–10 times, slowly.

BASIC PLIÉ

This move uses your buttocks and thighs, which makes it a great lower-body toner. When you do the move remember only to bend as far as you comfortably can before you lift your heels off the floor.

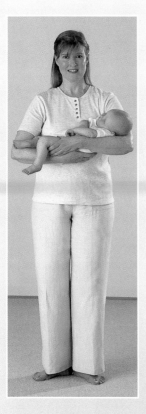

2 Maintain the squeeze on your buttocks as you bend your legs slowly. Concentrate on keeping your legs turned out and keeping your knees over the line of your toes. Then slowly straighten your legs again and come back to standing. Do 8 controlled pliés. Shake your legs out to relax them when you have finished the exercise.

1 Stand with your legs together and your feet slightly turned out so you can get the movement to start from the top of your legs. Squeeze your buttocks and turn your legs out from the top of your thighs.

85

Your postnatal check

Some doctors offer ongoing care in the days and weeks following the birth up to the postnatal check-up. Most postnatal check-ups happen at approximately six weeks after birth although it can be later if an IUD is to be fitted or a pap smear done. The purpose of the appointment is to check the physical and psychological health and well-being of the mother and to answer any questions that you might have.

Physical examination

These check-ups vary in their attention to detail, but your doctor is likely to be quite thorough, as he or she needs to make sure that you have recovered from the pregnancy and birth, both physically and emotionally. Your blood pressure will be taken to check that it is normal and your urine may be tested to ensure there is no infection. The incision scar will be examined to see that it has healed, and your abdomen will be felt to see if your uterus is reducing in size and shrinking back into the pelvic cavity.

Your weight may be checked, and if you are concerned about any increase, ask for advice on losing weight safely (see page 64).

You may be checked for haemorrhoids and your legs examined for swellin and potential varicose veins. You may be asked if you have any muscle pain and be given suggestions for caring for your back, especially if you suffered from

An all-round check-up
This is a good time for you to discuss with your caregiver any concerns you may have about your recovery.

> *I needed the doctor to explain why I'd had the operation*
>
> Julia *27 years*

I had to have an emergency acesarean and I felt really cheated about not being able to have the birth we'd planned. I couldn't talk about my feelings because I was sure no one would understand. I felt that my caregivers were to blame in some way. When I went for my postnatal check, the doctor explained exactly why I'd had to have a ceasarean and how the operation had saved my baby's life. For the first time I was able to accept what had happened. Now I am just glad that my baby is here, safe and well.

back problems during your pregnancy. Your breasts will be examined only if you have a particular concern.

You also may be asked about how breastfeeding is progressing, your future plans, and current sleep and feeding patterns. If yu are not immune to rubella and not given an immunisation before you left hospital, you will be offered one now. It's a good idea to have a list of any questions or concerns you have in these areas that you would like to raise – particularly if another caesarean will be needed should you have a subsequent baby and a form of contraception.

Psychological issues

Part of the postnatal assessment is likely to focus on emotional issues. Your caregiver may ask you to fill in a questionnaire related to your feelings and you may be asked about any baby blues symptoms. If depression is an issue, your doctor may prescribe an antidepressant of some sort to help you overcome these feelings and work with you to help you get whatever other suppoort you need.

This is a good time for you to discuss relationship issues, coping strategies and a return-to-work plan. Don't be afraid to ask about anything you feel unsure about, or to voice any concerns you may have. Your doctor is there to listen and to help you.

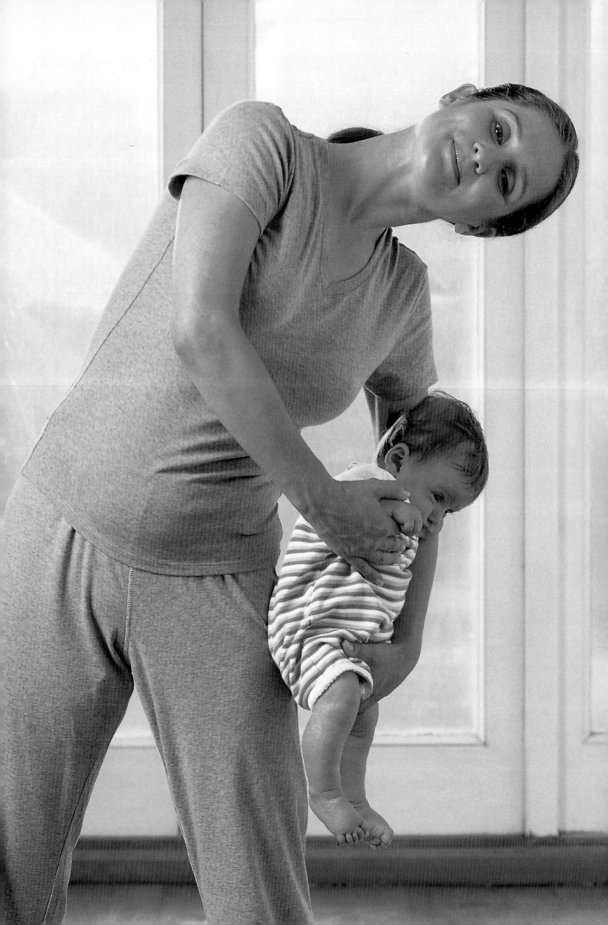

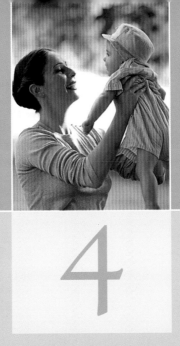

4

Weeks 13–24

Once you have had your postnatal check and you've been told that everything is returning to normal, you know you're well on the way to making a full recovery. Now you need to work on your exercise regime, gradually building on the exercises you have been doing over the past three months. Your baby will enjoy helping you with some of these, and you'll find that he or she makes an effective weight.

Weeks 13–24

Now that you have had your postnatal check-up with your healthcare provider and you are adjusting to your new life – life plus baby – you will likely feel comfortable increasing your fitness regime a little. Remember, your aim is to get yourself as strong and fit as you can now, while you have the time to exercise.

Good foundations

Although the first months with a new baby are all-absorbing and extremely tiring, it is also a good time to lay down the foundations of your fitness routine. You will be tired because of the interrupted sleep and constant demands, but there may also be times – even just half hours – when you can grab some time to yourself. Don't worry about cleaning the house, but do fit in 10 minutes of exercise. You will find that even this small amount of exercise will de-stress and re-energise you. These exercise sessions also will start to build some good muscle tone, which will stand you in good stead when your baby becomes a toddler and you have to chase after him.

Along with more complicated stomach work, you are now ready to do more intense toning moves. These moves, once learned, can then also be inserted into periods of cardiovascular exercise to increase your heart rate and the intensity of the routine.

Cardiovascular (CV) exercise

One of the things you can start to work on now is getting a little cardiovascular work in. Cardiovascular exercise simply means the kind of exercise you do when you feel the large muscles of the body working hard and your breathing rate goes up so that you can hear yourself puffing. Think of these simple routines as practice for the longer CV sessions that you can do when you're back to normal fitness.

CREATE YOUR OWN DANCE ROUTINE

Put on one of your favourite pieces of lively music. Now simply start to dance around a little. The more inspiring music you pick, the more energetically you will dance, so line up the CDs that you really enjoy.

Getting in the mood

Holding your baby close to your body, bend your knees and sway to pick up the rhythm. As you get more adventurous, waltz or twirl up and down the living room. Once you have warmed up, you can add in a grapevine step: step to side, step behind, step to the side, then step together. Continue doing the grapevine for a few minutes.

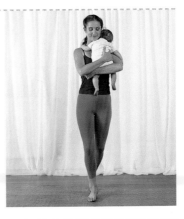

Box step

Now add in a box step: step forward on the right, then forward on the left, bending your knees a lot and pushing your hips forward as you move. Then step back on the right and back on the left. Do this for a few more minutes and then alternate with the grapevine.

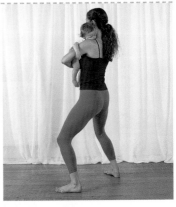

Jumping jacks

You should have really got into the swing of things by now and be ready to add some jumps to your moves. Support your baby's head and hold her close as you jump one leg out to one side and then back in again. Repeat on both sides. Now, add in a scissors jumping move: do the same as the sideways steps, but jump one foot forward and one foot behind, then jump to the opposite foot, forward and back. When you get tired, try marching on the spot.

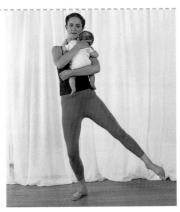

OBLIQUE STOMACH WORK

You can now begin to up the intensity of your stomach exercises. When you add twists and reaches to your stomach curls, you are bringing in the oblique muscles that wrap round the sides of your torso and support your back.

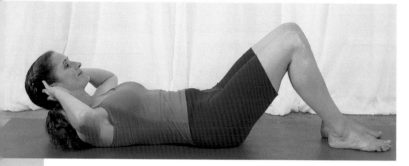

1 Lie on your back with your knees bent. Place your hands behind your head and lift up.

2 Now twist your head, shoulders and elbows (using the oblique muscles to twist) to the right.

3 Untwist and then twist to the other side. Untwist to the front and lower your upper body down to the floor. Perform this move (lift up, twist, untwist, twist to the other side, untwist and lower to the floor) 8 times.

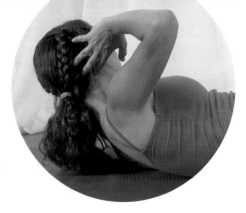

TWIST AND STRETCH

This is another stomach exercise that will work your oblique muscles. If you feel any pulling around the caesarean scar when you do this exercise, stop immediately. Leave it for a day or two and then try again.

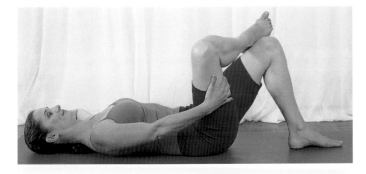

1 Lie with your left foot on the floor. Place your right leg across your knee, with your right ankle resting against your thigh. Wrap your right arm around your thigh and place your left arm behind your head.

2 Lift your head and shoulders and pull on your right arm to press your upper body diagonally across. Your aim is to press your left armpit toward your right knee. Keep your ankle resting on your thigh. Lie back and then repeat on the other side. Do 10 repetitions on each side, then repeat.

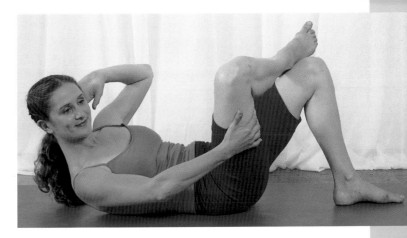

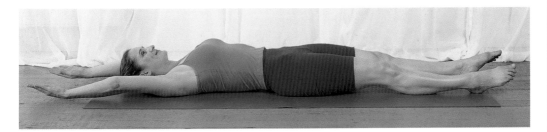

3 When you have finished stay lying down and do a full body stretch, stretching from your fingers right through to your toes.

BASIC LUNGE

This will help to work your thighs and calves. You may find it difficult to keep your balance as you step forward and then bend. Make sure that you always do the move slowly and with control.

1 Start with your arms out in front of you and take your left leg forward.

2 Now bend your knee and go into the lunge, keeping your weight balanced equally on both your legs so that your inner thighs are working. Make sure that your front knee is not over-shooting your toes because this can put pressure on the knee joint. Perform 10 of these moves on each leg.

JUMP LUNGE

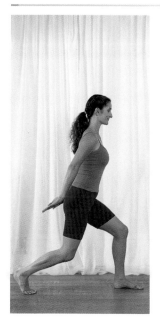

1 When you are confident with the basic lunge, step into the lunge and hold the position. Now bend your knees further and then push with your legs.

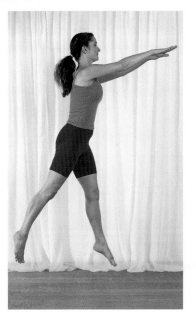

2 Bring your arms forward as you are propelled into the air. When you land make sure you bend your knees. Repeat 8 times on each forward leg.

SCISSORS LUNGE

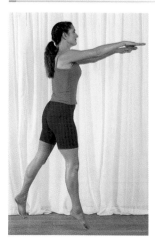

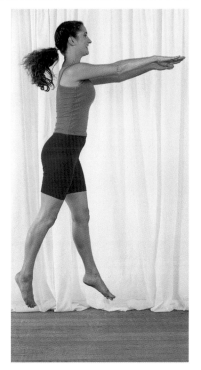

2 Change legs (the front one goes back and the back one comes forward) and then land with bent knees as before. To perform this move well you need to really propel yourself into the air and swap your legs at the last moment. Try 5 jumps with each leg in front.

1 Assume the basic lunge position and bend your knees further. Now push off into the air – try to suspend yourself for a moment.

Exercises for you and your baby

In your quest for continuing fitness and health, you need to exercise regularly. You may find that your baby is awake more now, so you could include her in your exercise sessions. Below are some great toning exercises that you can do while holding your baby. Think of your baby as an ever-increasing weight – as she gets bigger and stronger so do you because you are lifting more kilos.

DANCE AND CUDDLE

This is a good warm-up exercise, and in a warm room it may even get you sweating. It's great to do it to music. Your arms may ache as you carry your baby around, but this just means you are toning them, too.

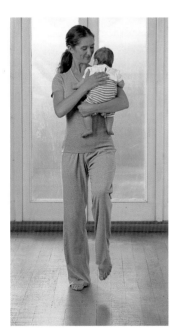

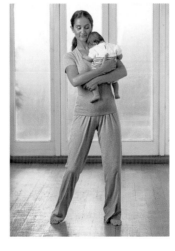

2 Step to one side and then step to the other.

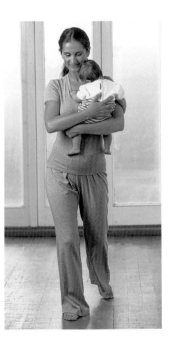

1 Start to move round the room with your baby in your arms. Lift your knees and march up and down.

3 Now move forward and back with your baby and if you're really getting into the rhythm, lift her up high as you come forward and pull him back in toward you as you step back. Do this routine for 4–5 minutes.

HOLD AND REACH

Once you have done your warm-up with the previous exercise, you can try something more energetic. As long as you are holding your baby securely, she should enjoy the movement.

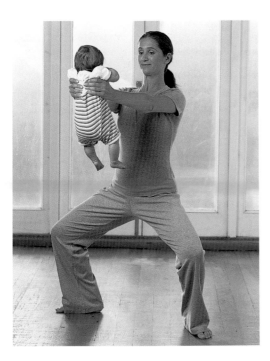

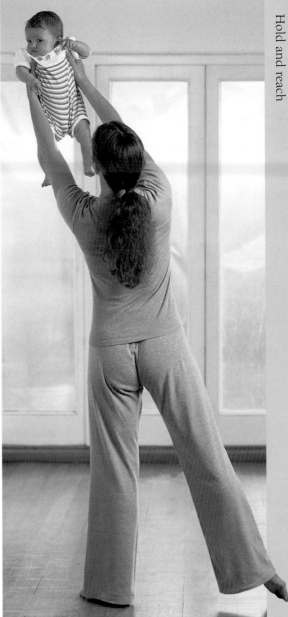

1 With your baby facing toward you, take hold of her under both arms. Hold her out at arms' length in front of you and bend both your knees.

2 From here, push up to one side and reach your baby up to the ceiling, holding her securely under her arms. Pull her back into your chest as you bend both knees again and then lift her up to the other side. Perform 8 of these on each side until you feel really warm.

BEND AND TWIST

This will tone your thigh muscles (*quadriceps*) as you bend and your waist (*oblique*) muscles as you twist. As you twist, make sure you keep your knees turned out and your hips straight. You should be twisting from your upper body.

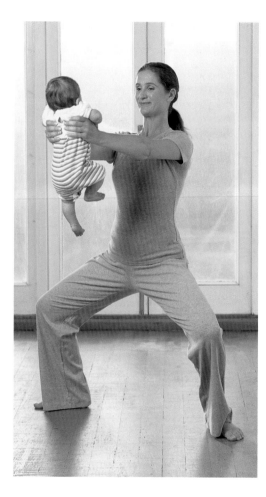 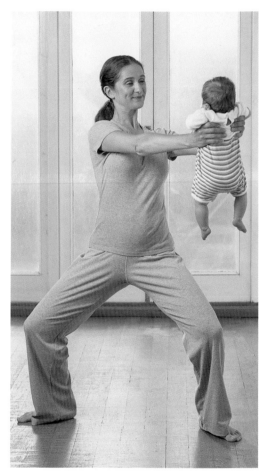

1 The best way to hold your baby for this move is under both her arms. Now turn your feet out and place them wide apart. Bend your knees slowly, pressing your knees out over your toes.

2 When your knees are well bent, pull in your stomach muscles and use them to twist and swing your baby round to one side, then round to the other. As you bend, be sure your knees are following the line of your toes. Straighten your legs and repeat. Perform 8–10 of these moves; your baby should enjoy the swinging sensation.

THIGH SHAPER

This is a great exercise for really working and shaping your thighs, and your baby will add an additional toning effect. You will feel the work in the front of your thigh as you extend and bend your leg.

2 Extend your bent leg (the one the baby is sitting on) and hold the extension for 3 seconds. Then bend your leg back in again. Keep your abdominals tight when you do this exercise to support your torso, and keep your supporting leg pulled up – don't sink into your hip when you are on one leg. Perform 8 extensions and then repeat with your other leg.

1 Stand with your back to a wall and bend one knee up in front of you. Now place your baby astride your knee and hold her against your body to give her support.

SIDE STRENGTHENER

The action of leaning over will stretch out your side, and by contracting the muscles on the opposite side as you come up, you will strengthen these muscles as you lift your baby back up again.

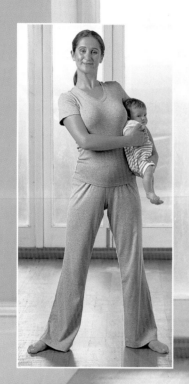

1 Stand with your feet wide apart and knees slightly bent and hold your baby to one side of you. The best hold for this is to place one arm down the front of your baby's body and hold her under her bottom, between her legs. With your other arm you can steady her by holding under her arm. Press her into your hip for further support.

2 Now lean to the side. Let your head, shoulders and rib cage lean as the weight of your baby pulls you into a side bend. Think about contracting the muscles on the opposite side of your stomach as you come back to an upright position. Perform 8 leans on each side.

PERSONAL PUSH-UP

Now get down on all fours over your baby. You can have a little chat with her while you check you have equal weight on both hands and knees. Make sure your shoulders are in line with your hands before you begin.

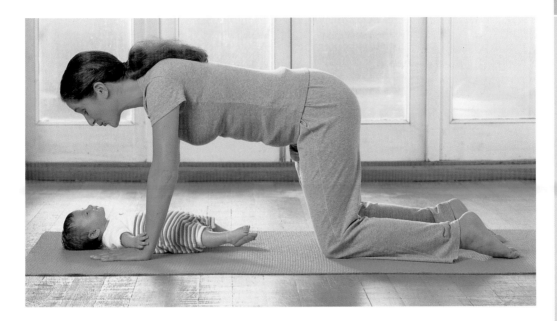

1 Bend your arms so that you lower your face down toward your baby, maintaining eye contact the whole time. She will love it.

2 As you lower your body, keep your back straight. It is important to get your shoulders over your hands as you lower with your elbows, pressing out to the sides as you bend. Perform this move 10 times. If you get low enough you can give baby a kiss at the bottom of the move.

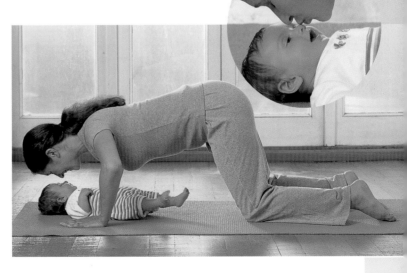

101

STOMACH TIGHTENER

You also can involve your baby when you are doing your stomach exercises. You will feel this movement in your abdominals. As you get stronger you can inch your baby further up your chest to provide even more resistance.

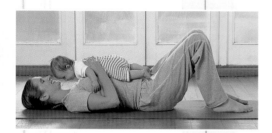

1 Lie on your back with knees bent and place your baby along your rib cage. Hold her upright with your hands as you curl your head and shoulders off the floor.

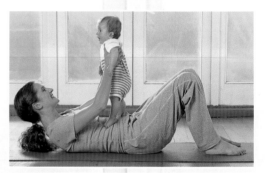

2 Concentrate on lifting your head and shoulders as high off the floor as you can. Hold at the top of the move momentarily and then rest back down.

3 Do 10 repetitions. Rest briefly, and then sit up and lift your baby high in the air.

BOTTOM BOOSTER

This exercise will work your buttock (gluteal) muscles. Your baby should be very impressed with the ride she gets as you lift and lower your hips. As with all these exercises, as your baby gets heavier, the resistance increases.

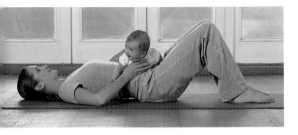
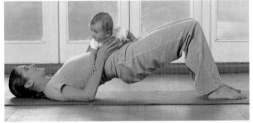

1 Lie on your back with your knees bent and place your baby across your hips, holding her steady with your hands.

2 Now, squeezing your buttocks, lift your hips up into the air. Perform 10 repetitions of this exercise.

STRETCH OUT

Finish off your workout together by playing a little game with your baby. This will stretch your legs and the sides of your stomach and waist, which is an important part of cooling down.

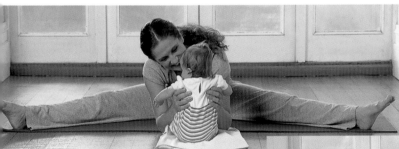

1 Holding your baby under her arms, sit down with your legs open and reach forward as far as you can.

2 Now lie her down and keep changing your position so that you have to stretch in different directions to reach her. This will give you a good stretch all over.

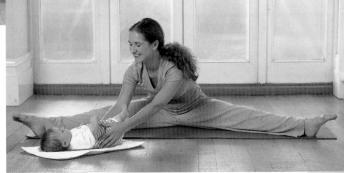

Walking and jogging

The best thing about this type of exercise is that you and your baby can do it together, whenever you feel like it. All you need is a pavement, a park or an open space where you can walk briskly, knowing that you are both benefitting from the fresh air and the exercise.

Out and about
The movement and the closeness make a baby carrier a treat for both your baby and you.

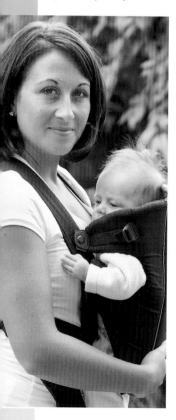

Walking

When you first go out walking with your baby you will probably find it easiest to walk with her in her buggy. Don't overdo it by trying to walk too far or too fast at first. Take her out each day, starting off walking briskly for ten minutes, and then gradually over several weeks increase the amount of time until you have reached 30 minutes. You are aiming to achieve a brisk 30-minute walk, at least three times a week.

Once you're comfortable with this, you may want to be more adventurous, perhaps going on a gentle hike out in the countryside. This is where a baby carrier will be useful. A carrier also has the advantage that both you and your partner can take turns walking with your baby.

Walk-jog

Now that you have got into the swing of walking briskly with your buggy, you may like to include some jogging for variety. As long as your body is up to the extra impact that running places on your joints, you can include a walk-jog technique into your regular exercise program. Start by running for just one minute, then walk for a while, and run again when you feel like it. Once you feel up to it, you can try running between two points such as lampposts or trees, and then walking between the next two, alternating until you have had enough. Keep up a good pace without overdoing it, and always include a cool-down period at the end of your walk-jog session.

Whether you are walking or jogging, always wear comfortable footwear that will give your feet ample support.

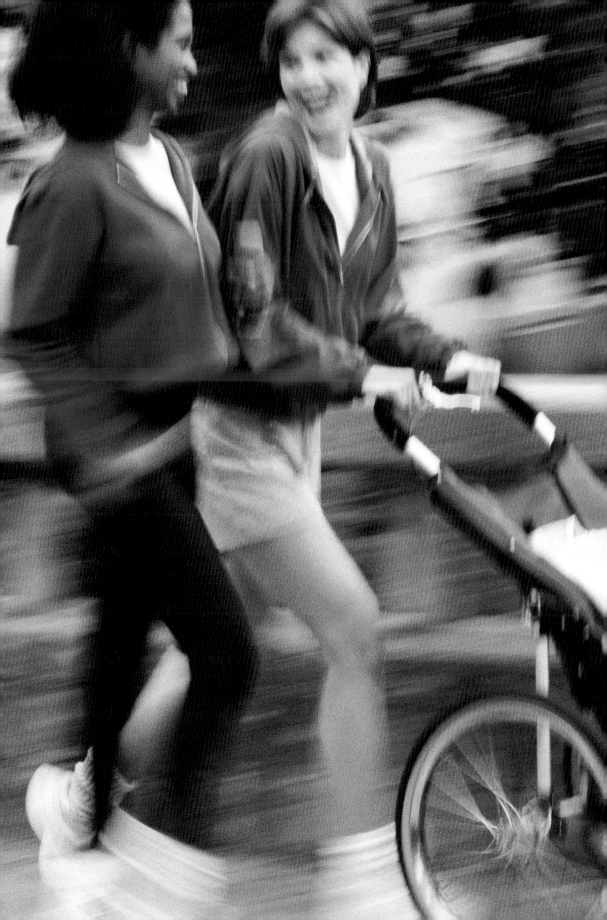

QUAD STRETCHES

Stretching is an important part of every exercise routine. The following stretches should be done after every exercise session, even if you have only been to the park. Here you can use your buggy as support.

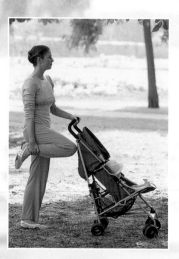

1 Stand with one hand on your baby's buggy and lift one foot up behind you. Take hold of your foot with your free hand and pull your heel toward your buttock.

2 Stand tall and pull in on your abdominals as you tilt your hips slightly forward. Hold the stretch for 10 seconds and then shake your leg out. Repeat with your other leg.

HAMSTRING STRETCH

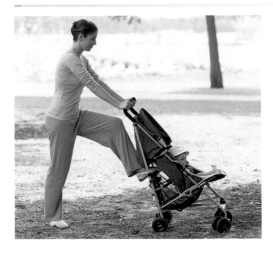

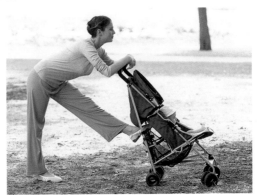

1 Take hold of the handle of your buggy and place one foot on the edge of the back of the seat.

2 Holding on with both hands and leaning back slightly, straighten your leg by pushing against the buggy. Hold this position for a few seconds then bend your leg back in. Repeat on the other side.

BACK STRETCH

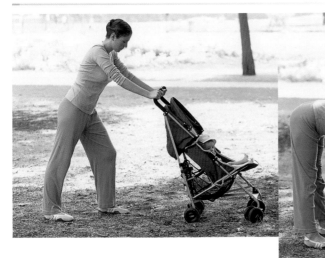

1 Hold the handles with both hands and push the buggy away from you. As you do this, keep your legs nearly straight and let the buggy pull your upper body forward.

2 When you reach a right-angle shape hold this stretch for 15 seconds. Then contract your abdominals as you stand up, pulling the buggy back toward you.

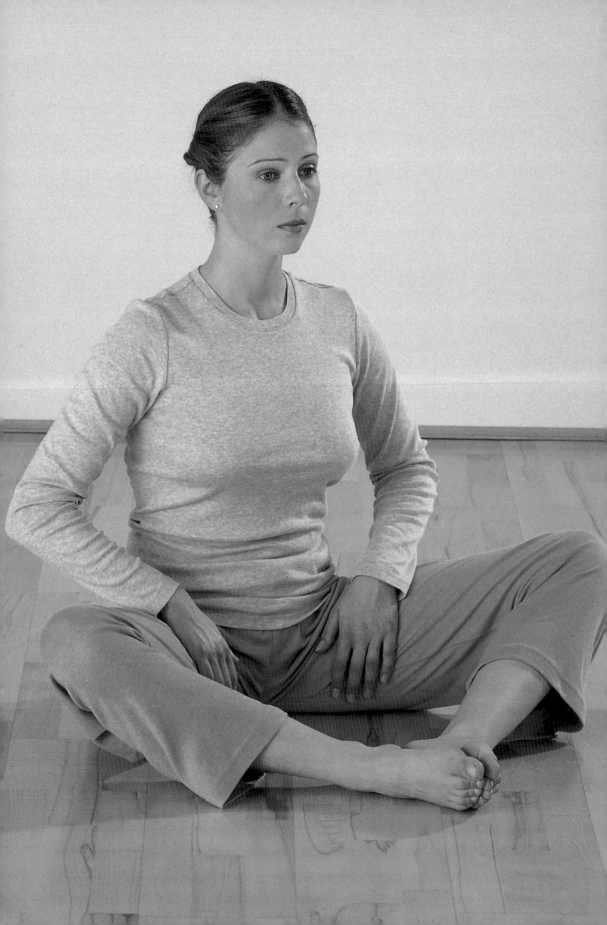

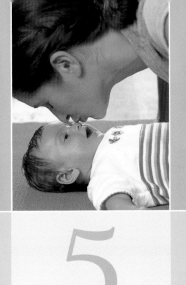

5

Return to normal

Six months after your operation you should be feeling almost like your old self again. You may have returned to your pre-pregnancy exercise regime, or perhaps you're happier continuing with the exercises you've been doing through your recovery period. The important thing is to build on your program and continue exercising on a regular basis. Your baby should now have settled into a routine, so there should be more time for you to relax and get in touch with your emotions.

Your pelvic floor

During pregnancy, pressure from the growing uterus can make the pelvic floor muscles stretched and weak. The pelvic floor is a very important area that needs working on, just as other muscles in the body need re-toning. Pelvic floor, or Kegel, exercises can be started soon after birth.

How it works

The pelvic floor is a sling of muscle which spans out and forms the bottom of the pelvis. The muscle is actually in two halves, with your vaginal, urinary and anal openings in the middle, and with the muscles attaching to the pubic bones in the front and to the coccyx (the bottom part of the spine) at the back. There are two layers of muscle: one superficial and the other deep. These muscles not only keep all openings closed off while supporting the weight of the internal organs but they also help with defaecation, sexual intercourse and the pushing out of the baby during childbirth. Keeping these muscles toned so that they contract and release strongly is of the utmost importance.

The effects of pregnancy

Pregnancy is a time when a woman tends to become much more aware of her pelvic floor and just how good a job it does. But you will also find that it needs encouragement, in the form of exercise, to keep it in good condition, because pregnancy may cause it some problems.

Because humans, as opposed to animals, carry their offspring in an upright position during pregnancy, the relatively weak muscles of the pelvic floor undergo constant pressure and the back does extra work. Along with this there are all sorts of hormonal, physiological and chemical changes which take place during pregnancy, including increased blood volume, fat stores being laid down and fluid retention, all of which put additional pressure on the pelvic floor. One of the major hormonal changes that takes place is the increase of relaxin hormone, which, as its name

Pelvic floor muscles
These muscles should be exercised before, during and after pregnancy.

> ❝ *I didn't think I needed to do pelvic floor exercises* ❞
>
> Anna 31 years
>
> *Because I'd been told early on in my pregnancy that I would be having my baby by caesarean I didn't think pelvic floor exercises would be important so I didn't bother to do them. After the birth I was so sore and uncomfortable, contracting those muscles was the last thing on my mind. How I wish now that I had! My daughter, Suzie, is nearly three years old and I still have problems with urinary incontinence. Sneezing, laughing and coughing are the worst.*

suggests, helps to relax all fibres in the body in order to allow the baby to pass through the pelvis.

You may have assumed that you wouldn't have problems with your pelvic floor because you had a caesarean. As the baby wasn't pushed out vaginally, the area will not have been overstretched. While this is true, and is certainly a benefit, this does not mean you can ignore your pelvic floor muscles. By the time of birth your pelvic floor will have been well and truly softened, whether the baby is passed out vaginally or not.

Possible problems

Weak and overstretched muscles can lose their reflex ability for sudden contraction and this can lead to a problem with urine leakage – more commonly known as stress incontinence. The bladder muscles do not seem to exercise the same control as they once had. Mild problems of this nature are actually quite common, with as many as one in three women suffering some form of leakage. Exercising the pelvic floor muscles before, during and after pregnancy can help to keep these muscles toned and supple so that they have more resistance to being stretched during childbirth and are more likely to rehabilitate faster.

Pelvic floor exercises

You should do your pelvic floor exercises from day one of your recovery. Because they can be done anywhere – standing up, in bed or sitting on a chair – it's easy to do them every day. Like all the muscles in your body, your pelvic floor muscles respond to work, so the more you persevere with these exercises the greater control you will have over these muscles.

Start gently

When you first try to get in touch with your pelvic floor, you may find it easier to get into a kneeling or an on all-fours position. Once you are in a comfortable position, try to draw the muscles up inside you, as if you were sucking something up into your body. You will find that your pelvic muscles respond like every other muscle in your body to being contracted and released.

Regular practice
Once you have learned to contract these muscles you can exercise them anywhere, at any time.

As you do this exercise nothing else in the body need move, so there should be no visible sign to anyone else that you are doing it, apart from an absorbed look on your face. You should definitely not hold your breath, even when you are just holding the contraction for a few seconds.

Because no one can see you doing these exercises you can practice contracting your pelvic floor muscles anywhere, any time, day or night. Once you feel confident about contracting and releasing your pelvic floor you should move on to the more advanced exercises on the opposite page.

Kegel method

This really works the pelvic floor and will tone and strengthen the muscles if you do the exercise regularly.

Contract and release your pelvic floor while breathing normally, but start to hold for longer. The Kegel method involves building up to holds of 20 seconds – which can seem like quite a long time – in order to really work those muscles and tone them. Don't forget to stay relaxed and keep breathing normally. You can also vary the speed. Try contracting them in time to music! Do short holds and then longer ones. Practise for 2–3 minutes at a time.

Back, middle, front

Once you are able to hold the exercise for several minutes at a time, you can work on the separate rings of muscle involved.

As you become more aware and gain greater control over your muscles you can try experimenting a little. There are actually three rings of muscle which surround each of the openings, and each band of muscle is actually capable of being contracted in isolation. Try to squeeze the muscles around the back passage (anus) then release. Now try and squeeze the muscles around the vagina (the muscles you use during sex) and release. Finally, squeeze the muscles you use when you go to the toilet to pass urine and release. Practise "back, middle and front" until you have gained full control over each individual ring of muscle. Now try and hold each band of muscle for one minute before releasing and moving on to the next. Do several sets of this exercise at least three times a day.

Posture pointers

Whenever you are standing, if you can keep your posture good then you will be toning your stomach muscles and protecting your back from extra strain. You can work on your posture by using the neutral spine alignment whenever you lie down, and the coccyx-down alignment whenever you are standing.

Lying correctly

When you lie down on the floor to do any exercise, before you begin try to adopt a neutral spine position. You can achieve this by bending your knees and tilting your pelvis so that your lower back is pressed flat against the floor. Once you're in this position relax a little so that your spine comes away from the floor. There should now be a gap between the floor and your spine, but not an over-emphasised one. This position puts your spine in neutral alignment, which is the safest position when performing sit-ups and other prone exercises.

POSTURE PERFECTER

You can check your posture is correct by doing the following:

O *Stand against a wall with your feet flat on the floor*

O *Press your lower back flat against the wall until you feel your stomach muscles engaging to hold the tilt of your pelvis*

O *Lift the rest of your body upward so that you feel as if your head is pressing up through the ceiling*

O *Press your shoulders down behind you*

O *Drop your chin slightly so that your neck is elongated*

O *Once you have absorbed this stance, take one step away from the wall and try to relax into the position*

Standing tall

If you are standing correctly you should feel a lengthening through your body with your head pressing upward, while your coccyx or tail bone is being pulled downward. This coccyx-down alignment can be practised anywhere – standing at the bus stop or in a queue. While you are still recovering from your caesarean section, you may find that it helps to use your baby's buggy for support.

Once you are comfortable with this position you should be able to adapt it so that you automatically "walk tall" when you are out and about. If you are pushing your baby in his buggy, you will need to concentrate on your posture to make sure that you don't hunch forward over the handles.

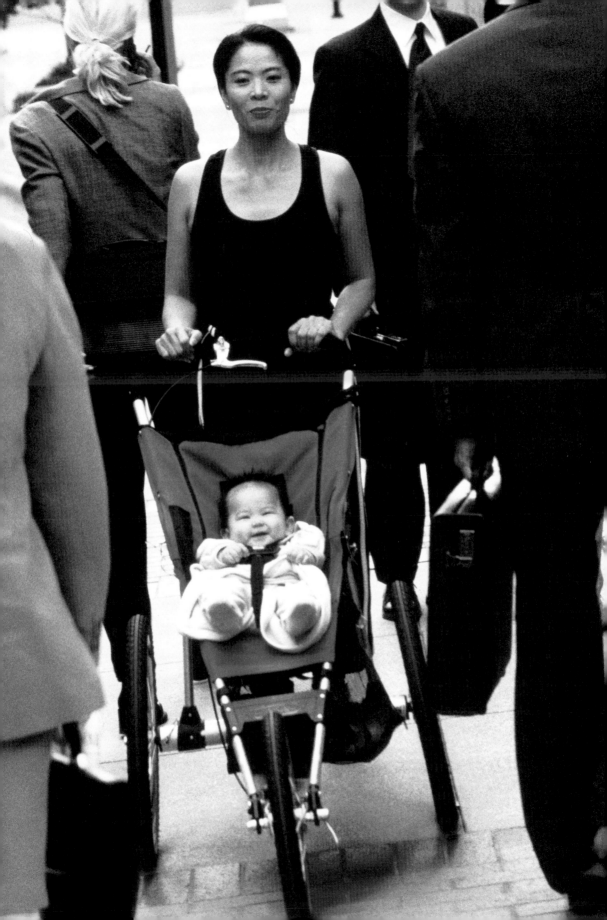

How to build your program

Although the old cliché is true – that life will never be the same again – you will get used to a new kind of life that will be all the richer because of your baby. It is also true that your figure may never be the same again – this doesn't mean your figure will look worse, it could well be better.

A realistic approach

It can take a year, or even longer, before you feel truly back to your old levels of energy and fitness. It can take even longer if your baby is not a good sleeper, leaving you tired all the time. Physically your shape may have changed, for example your waist measurement may be quite a lot bigger. This could be due to the lasting effects of the hormone, relaxin, expanding the rib cage or to some of the excess weight you gained during pregnancy. If you still have a bit of a belly, don't worry. As long as you keep working on the stomach muscles and your general fitness, this will improve. Be aware of your posture, too, whenever you stand, practise standing tall. Try to pull up off your spine and pull in on your abdominals.

Your recovery
You'll be amazed at how much stronger and fitter you have become since you first came home.

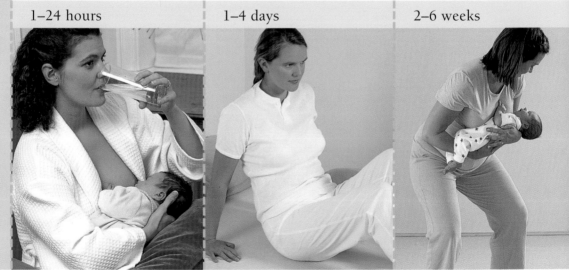

1–24 hours   1–4 days   2–6 weeks

Occasional twinges

You may also find that your scar twinges from time to time – this can happen years after the birth, but as long as all you are feeling is mild discomfort rather than actual physical pain you need not be alarmed by this.

Weight gain

You may find you have a tendency to gain weight around your stomach and back area because your body is still in pregnancy mode. Keep working on your fitness regime and you will eventually manage to get rid of this excess weight.

Bear in mind tht recovery from a caesarean section takes time, so don't beat yourself up if you haven't lost all your extra weight in the first four months or if you still don't feel on top of the world. Pace yourself and build up slowly – you will get there, eventually.

KEEP UP THE GOOD WORK

In order to keep the improvements in your fitness going:

○ *Try to put aside some time every other day to exercise*

○ *Your workout routine doesn't need to take long. If 10 minutes is all you have then still do it – even 10 minutes will make a difference*

○ *Exercise along with your baby – use the buggy for a workout (see page 106) or use him as a weightl (see page 96)*

○ *Whenever you can, walk. Take the buggy, put your baby in a sling and practise fast-walking. Swing your arms so that you can feel you are working hard.*

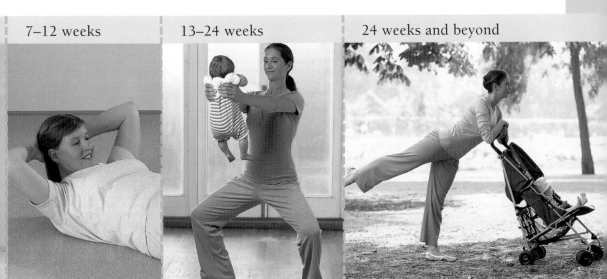

7–12 weeks | 13–24 weeks | 24 weeks and beyond

Learn to relax

As well as exercising regularly you also need to find time to relax. Start by setting aside a few moments' relaxation a day. The 5-minute relaxer described opposite is ideal for incorporating into your exercise routine or you can opt for something that's more personally pleasing – such as a solitary bath.

Relaxing activities

If the only place you can get five minutes on your own is in the bathroom, then go there and lock the door. Even if you can only grab half an hour once a week for a luxurious soak, it can make a difference to your overall feeling of well-being. Get someone else to look after your baby, light some candles, play soothing music and pour some of your favourite bath oil into warm water. Then lie back, shut your eyes and relax for as long as you can. Try to empty your mind so that all you are thinking about is what you are doing with your body and nothing else.

Sometimes a change of scenery can give you a lift, so think about arranging a night out with your friends, or hire a baby-sitter and spend a romantic evening with your partner. You may feel too tired to be bothered when you've been looking after your baby all day, but if you make the effort, you'll be surprised at how good you feel afterward.

If a lack of sleep is getting you down, work out with your partner ways of getting some extra sleep. Perhaps he could look after your baby in the mornings on the weekend so that you can have a lie-in, or maybe he could do some of the housework so that you can nap when your baby is sleeping. You'll be amazed at the difference an extra hour or two in bed can make. You'll find that you are much more able to manage after a good sleep.

RELAXING OILS

Add a few drops of one of these essential oils to an almond oil base for bathing.

○ *Frankincense has the ability to slow down and deepen breathing*
○ *Geranium will relieve nervous tension and stress*
○ *Lavender balances both mind and body and induces sleep*
○ *Mandarin is the gentlest of all oils and will relieve insomnia and nervous tension*

5-minute relaxer

For this to work you need to empty your mind and concentrate on your body, so it's best to do this when your baby is asleep or is being looked after by someone else.

Lie on your back on the floor of a warm room and concentrate on your breathing for a few minutes. Listen to your breath going in and out of your body. Now concentrate on your body, starting with your head, and try to relax each part.

First, press your head into the floor and then release it. Feel your neck muscles ease and note how your head is fully supported on the floor. Try to register how your head is heavy and your neck is soft. Now press your shoulders toward the floor and release. Note again the changes in your muscles as you use them and then relax them.

Work your way down the body doing the same for each part. Once you have reached your feet, lie there and evaluate. Note where your body touches the floor and where it doesn't. Check the position of your hands and your feet – are they equal? (If they aren't it doesn't matter, it's simply a question of noticing.)

To bring yourself back to reality, slowly point your feet and tense your lower leg muscles as you stretch your legs. Lift your arms above your head and do the same stretch with your upper body. Take a deep breath in, roll onto your side and slowly come up to sitting.

Pamper yourself

If you can find the time, it's worth booking yourself a whole body massage or a reflexology session. Suggest this if anyone asks you what you would like for a gift. Massage of any form is a great tension reliever and will leave you feeling revived and your muscles invigorated. Alternatively, there are a number of treatments you can try yourself at home, such as the reviving self-massage shown opposite. If you are breastfeeding you should check that the oils you are going to use are suitable.

Home-made masks

You can create soothing treatments made from ingredients you probably already have at home. Combine 2 tablespoons of unpasteurised honey with 2 teaspoons of freshly squeezed lemon or lime juice, pat it on your face and neck for a moisturising treat, then wash it off with warm water after 15 minutes. Another refreshing mask calls for 2 tablespoons gram flour mixed with 1 tablespoon live natural yogurt and 6 drops of sandalwood essential oil. Massage this over your face avoiding your eyes and mouth and splash off with water after 10 minutes.

Treat your feet

Check your feet regularly for cuts, blisters or sores. Use a pumice stone to smooth away any corns or calluses. Wash them at the end of each day in warm, not hot, water and dry them well, particularly between the toes. You can keep the skin soft by applying body lotion to the tops and soles of your feet. Keep your toenails trimmed, cutting them straight across, using clippers not scissors, and smooth the edges with an emery board.

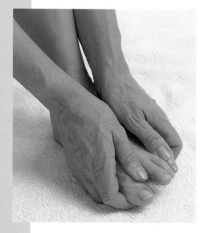

Revive tired feet
Gently massage the toes and arches of your feet using a little lotion to keep them soft.

My mum comes over once a week to look after my baby so that I can have a couple of hours to myself.

REVIVING SELF-MASSAGE

Make this even more delightful by using a massage oil made of a few drops of an uplifting essential oil such as geranium or peppermint in an almond base oil – rub the oil between your hands to warm it before you begin.

Starting with the head

The room where you are going to do your massage should be warm and draft-free. If possible, shut the door and dim any lights so that your surroundings are calm and peaceful. Start by tapping your fingers lightly over your scalp from front to back. Use firm pressure and continue to do this for two to three minutes, always working from the front to back of your head.

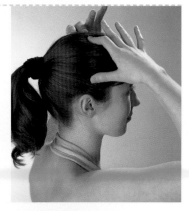

Working down your body

Make a loose fist with your left hand and pummel over your shoulder on the right side. Do this for two minutes and then change hands. Now pour a little oil into your palm and warm it between your hands. Briskly sweep your right hand down your left arm (from your shoulder to your fingertips), pulling off at the tips with an energizing shake of your wrist. Repeat several times. Switch hands.

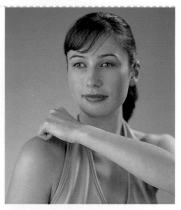

Finishing off

Now, with your right hand make kneading movements down the left side of your neck, across your shoulder and down your upper arm. Repeat on your right side. Moving downward, pummel your buttocks with soft, loose fists. Then, using the sides of your hands, bounce them up and down over the fronts and sides of your thighs in a chopping motion. Finally, pummel your chest with soft, loose fists, letting out an "aaahhh" cry.

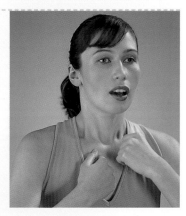

Repeat caesareans

In the past 35 years the caesarean rate has greatly increased in the US, Canada and the UK, yet the World Health Organisation maintains that no region in the world is justified in having a caesarean rate greater than 10 percent while rates above 15 percent do more harm than good.

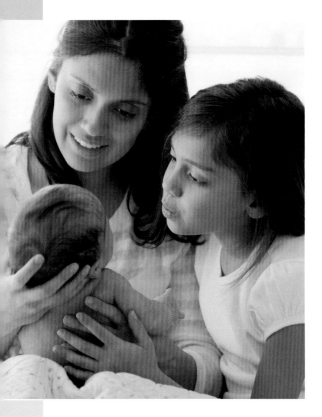

Vaginal birth
Even if your first child was born by caesarean, it may be possible for you to have subsequent vaginal deliveries.

The reasons for a rising rate

Some caesarean prevention organisations have become concerned that C-sections are being done too routinely, and not always for the benefit of mother and baby. Research has disproved the ideas that more mothers are asking for the procedure and that the number of women who genuinely need a caesarean is rising. Instead, among the main factors responsible, is the low priority given to enhancing a woman's own abilities to give birth, the side effects of common labour interventions such as induction and fetal monitoring, ignorance of the possible harms of the procedure coupled with a tolerance of surgery even when not medically needed.

The facts of the matter

Elective caesareans are not without risk. For the baby, premature birth and respiratory distress syndrome may occur. For the mother, there may be a delayed opportunity to interact with or breastfeed her newborn in addition to a possibility of infection, surgical injury, adhesions and blood clots.

One of the reasons for the high number of caesareans is that many mothers are concerned as to whether they can attempt a normal delivery once they have already had a caesarean; in the UK, 29 percent of

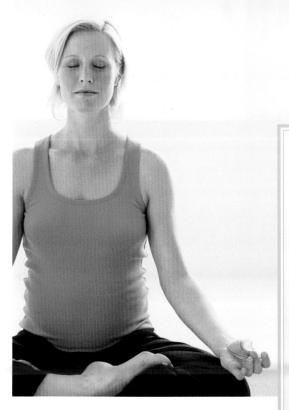

HOW TO PREVENT A CAESAREAN

Not all caesareans can or should be prevented, but the following situations are more likely to result in a vaginal delivery. A caesarean prevention organisation should be able to give you further advice.

* *Your hospital and/or your consultant's rate of caesareans is lower than average and your consultant is sympathetic to your cause.*
* *You are in top condition for labour and have an indeependent midwife.*
* *You have had a vaginal delivery or a successful VBAC in the past.*
* *Your prior caesarean was performed for a non-recurring cause, like a breech presentation or placenta praevia.*
* *Your prior caesarean was performed eiher prior to or early in labour (not after full dilatation).*
* *Your current labour occurs spontaneously, your waters break on their own and you are not put on a drip to speed labour up.*
* *Your baby's heartbeat is monitored regularly.*
* *You keep moving around and try to stay upright.*

caesareans are repeat caesareans. This is often because the mum is anxious that the problem that necessitated the first caesarean will recur, or the caregiver responsible for the birth thinks that because the woman had a caesarean already, having a second one is the easiest option.

But it is possible for a woman to have a vaginal birth after a caesarean (VBAC). In fact, around 60–80 percent of women who attempt VBAC succeed. However, there exists a small risk of uterine rupture and fetal death rates are slightly higher than with a repeat caesarean.

If you want to attempt a VBAC, it is important to find a consultant who will deliver you. You must have your baby in hospital so that any complications can be dealt with immediately. Your uterine contractions and your baby's heartbeat will be continually monitored and, if induction is necessary, you will given a medication that will not create uterine hyperstimulation.

Frequently asked questions

Although this book aims to cover everything you need to know when having a cesarean, there are always some questions that apply personally to you. Here are some of the most frequently asked questions with their answers, but if you need more information talk to your healthcare provider.

Is it true that the use of electronic fetal monitoring during labour is more likely to lead to a caesarean?
While fetal distress, the commonest cause of caesarean section, can be diagnosed by electronic fetal monitoring, often the machines give a faulty reading. If a technician or midwife believes that fetal distress is putting the baby at risk, he or she will often recommend a caesareane.

I've read about the psychological effects of a caesarean on the mother, but are there any similar effects on the child ?
Only a limited number of follow-up studies of infants born by caesarean have been done, but these show no evidence of adverse psychological effects on the children concerned.

I have been told that I will need to have a caesarean and I am a real coward when it comes to pain. Although I don't feel too concerned about the operation itself because, I am worried about having the staples removed afterwards. When will this be done and will it hurt?
Staples are usually removed a few days after the operation, either before you leave hospital or in your

doctor's surgery once you have returned home. The removal is usually not painful, unless the staples have become embedded in the skin as the incision begins to heal. In this case, you may experience some discomfort when they are taken out, but this only lasts for a short time.

I would like to try for a VBAC instead of repeat caesarean but there seems to be conflicting information as to which is best. Why is ithis?

Up until the 1990s, a woman who had a caesarean section almost always had a planned repeat caesarean and not a VBAC for any subsequent births. Doctors were concerned that the scar from the past cut in the uterus could open during labour (uterine rupture), and cause serious complications. During the 25 years or so, however, many health professionals, advocates, policy makers and researchers encouraged VBAC in light of a change in location of the uterine cut to an area much less likely to open during labour and research establishing the safety of VBAC while highlighting c-section risks.Now the pendulum is swinging back from VBAC, with new calls for routine repeat caesareans. This reversal leaves many women with caesarean scars struggling to make sense of conflicting, incomplete and sometimes misleading information about VBAC vs. repeat caesareans.

I was surprised to have a bloody vaginal discharge after my operation. I though only women who'd had vaginal births would lose blood from their vaginas. Why does this still happen when you've had a caesarean and how long will it last?

Lochia is the vaginal discharge which is experienced by all women after giving birth. It comes from the site where the placenta was attached to the uterine wall, so the way your baby was born and how the placenta was delivered make no difference to the discharge. For the first week it is bright red; gradually turning to pink and then a yellowish-white, and it can last up to six weeks.

How soon after having a caesarean can I start swimming and using the gym again?

Most healthcare professionals suggest that women wait at least six weeks before returning to the gym. However, there is no reason why you can't start swimming again as soon as the lochia ceases – usually between four and six weeks after delivery.

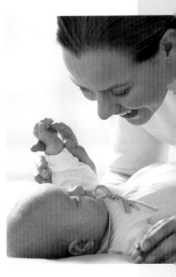

Index

Acknowledgments

Chrissie Gallagher-Mundy would like to thank her sons Killian and Fynn (both of whom were delivered by cesarean section), for kick-starting her interest in the subject, and all at Carroll and Brown for their professionalism and attention to detail.

Carroll & Brown Publishers would like to thank:

Production Karol Davies, Nigel Reed
IT Paul Stradling, Nicky Rein
Picture research Sandra Schneider
Photographic assistance David Yems
Hair and make-up Toka Hombu
Illustrations Amanda Williams
Proofreader Geoffrey West
Index Anna Amari-Parker

Thanks also to our mothers and babies:
Sandrine and Mila
Sue and Dean
Miriam and Celeste
Helen and Max
Jayne and Dalia
Sophy and Lily
Marissa and Teague

Picture credits

page 12	Simon Fraser/SPL
page 16	Frances Tout/Mother and Baby Picture Library
page 17	Photolibrary
page 18	Getty Images
page 20	Camera Press/Your Pregnancy
page 21	Frances Tout/Mother and Baby Picture Library
page 22	Powerstock
page 25	Powerstock
page 33	Perfectly Happy People Ltd
page 52	Getty Images
page 54	Gary D. Landsman/Corbis
page 56	Powerstock
page 86	Ian Hooton/Mother and Baby Picture Library
page 115	Powerstock

Thanks also to Perfectly Happy People Ltd (www.thebabycatalogue.com) *for their help.*